VOLUME ONE HUNDRED AND EIGHTEEN

ADVANCES IN PARASITOLOGY

Advances in Molecular and Automated Diagnosis of Intestinal Parasites of Animals and Humans

VOLUME ONE HUNDRED AND EIGHTEEN

ADVANCES IN PARASITOLOGY

Advances in Molecular and Automated Diagnosis of Intestinal Parasites of Animals and Humans

Edited by

LAURA RINALDI
Department of Veterinary Medicine and Animal Production, University of Naples "Federico II", Naples, Italy

GIUSEPPE CRINGOLI
Department of Veterinary Medicine and Animal Production, University of Naples "Federico II", Naples, Italy

ELSEVIER

ACADEMIC PRESS
An imprint of Elsevier

Academic Press is an imprint of Elsevier
125 London Wall, London EC2Y 5AS, United Kingdom
The Boulevard, Langford Lane, Kidlington, Oxford OX5 1GB, United Kingdom
50 Hampshire Street, 5th Floor, Cambridge, MA 02139, United States
525 B Street, Suite 1650, San Diego, CA 92101, United States

First edition 2022

Notices
Knowledge and best practice in this field are constantly changing. As new research and experience broaden our understanding, changes in research methods, professional practices, or medical treatment may become necessary.

Practitioners and researchers must always rely on their own experience and knowledge in evaluating and using any information, methods, compounds, or experiments described herein. In using such information or methods they should be mindful of their own safety and the safety of others, including parties for whom they have a professional responsibility.

To the fullest extent of the law, neither the Publisher nor the authors, contributors, or editors, assume any liability for any injury and/or damage to persons or property as a matter of products liability, negligence or otherwise, or from any use or operation of any methods, products, instructions, or ideas contained in the material herein.

ISBN: 978-0-323-99396-8
ISSN: 0065-308X

For information on all Academic Press publications
visit our website at https://www.elsevier.com/books-and-journals

Publisher: Zoe Kruze
Acquisitions Editor: Leticia Lima
Developmental Editor: Cindy Angelita Gardose
Production Project Manager: Abdulla Sait
Cover Designer: Mark Rogers

Typeset by STRAIVE, India

Contents

Contributors

Zeno Bisoffi
Department of Infectious Tropical diseases and Microbiology, IRCCS Sacro Cuore Don Calabria Hospital; Department of Diagnostics and Public Health, University of Verona, Verona, Italy

Richard S. Bradbury
School of Health and Life Sciences, Federation University Australia, Berwick, VC, Australia

Dora Buonfrate
Department of Infectious Tropical diseases and Microbiology, IRCCS Sacro Cuore Don Calabria Hospital, Verona, Italy

V. Castilla Gómez de Agüero
Instituto de Ganadería de Montaña (CSIC-Universidad de León), Departamento de Sanidad Animal, Facultad de Veterinaria, Universidad de León, León, Spain

J. Charlier
Kreavet, Kruibeke, Belgium

Giuseppe Cringoli
Department of Veterinary Medicine and Animal Production, University of Naples "Federico II", Naples, Italy

C. de Queiroz
Faculty of Veterinary Medicine, 3331 Hospital Drive, Host-Parasite Interactions (HPI) Program University of Calgary, Calgary, Alberta, Canada; Faculty of Veterinary Medicine, St Georges University, Grenada

J.S. Gilleard
Faculty of Veterinary Medicine, 3331 Hospital Drive, Host-Parasite Interactions (HPI) Program University of Calgary, Calgary, Alberta, Canada

J. Krücken
Institute for Parasitology and Tropical Veterinary Medicine, Veterinary Centre for Resistance Research, Freie Universität Berlin, Berlin, Germany

M. Martinez-Valladares
Instituto de Ganadería de Montaña (CSIC-Universidad de León), Departamento de Sanidad Animal, Facultad de Veterinaria, Universidad de León, León, Spain

M.P. Maurelli
Department of Veterinary Medicine and Animal Production, University of Naples "Federico II", Naples, Italy

Paola Paradies
Department of Emergency and Organs Transplantation, Veterinary Section, Campus of Veterinary Medicine, University of Bari, Bari, Italy

P. Pepe
Department of Veterinary Medicine and Animal Production, University of Naples "Federico II", Naples, Italy

Laura Rinaldi
Department of Veterinary Medicine and Animal Production, University of Naples "Federico II", Naples, Italy

Francesca Tamarozzi
Department of Infectious Tropical diseases and Microbiology, IRCCS Sacro Cuore Don Calabria Hospital, Verona, Italy

G. von Samson-Himmelstjerna
Institute for Parasitology and Tropical Veterinary Medicine, Veterinary Centre for Resistance Research, Freie Universität Berlin, Berlin, Germany

T. Wang
Kreavet, Kruibeke, Belgium

Matthew R. Watts
Centre for Infectious Diseases and Microbiology, Institute of Clinical Pathology and Medical Research – New South Wales Health Pathology and Sydney Institute for Infectious Diseases, Westmead Hospital, University of Sydney, Sydney, New South Wales, Australia

Preface

Diagnosis of gastrointestinal nematodes in animals and humans has been neglected for many years, and in the past too little investment has been made in developing and improving diagnostic tools, thus undermining the undoubted benefits of surveillance and control programs at various levels. However, a renewed impetus from the scientific community and the acceleration of technological innovations are leading to a renaissance of interest in developing diagnostic capacity for nematode infections in medical and veterinary parasitology.

The objective of this volume is to provide an overview of parasitological, immunological, and molecular tests for the diagnosis of two important groups of nematodes, i.e., *Strongyloides stercoralis,* which infects humans and dogs, and gastrointestinal nematodes, which infect livestock and companion animals.

Advances in diagnostic methods for these intestinal parasites are also presented, such as (i) automated artificial intelligence-based copromicroscopic methods, (ii) immunodiagnosis, and (iii) molecular- and proteome-based approaches.

We thank all the authors who kindly contributed to the preparation of this special volume, which highlights the importance of the diagnosis of nematodes with medical and veterinary relevance.

Laura Rinaldi and Giuseppe Cringoli

CHAPTER ONE

The diagnosis of human and companion animal *Strongyloides stercoralis* infection: Challenges and solutions. A scoping review

Dora Buonfrate[a],*, Francesca Tamarozzi[a], Paola Paradies[b], Matthew R. Watts[c], Richard S. Bradbury[d,†], and Zeno Bisoffi[a,e,†]

[a]Department of Infectious Tropical diseases and Microbiology, IRCCS Sacro Cuore Don Calabria Hospital, Verona, Italy
[b]Department of Emergency and Organs Transplantation, Veterinary Section, Campus of Veterinary Medicine, University of Bari, Bari, Italy
[c]Centre for Infectious Diseases and Microbiology, Institute of Clinical Pathology and Medical Research – New South Wales Health Pathology and Sydney Institute for Infectious Diseases, Westmead Hospital, University of Sydney, Sydney, New South Wales, Australia
[d]School of Health and Life Sciences, Federation University Australia, Berwick, VC, Australia
[e]Department of Diagnostics and Public Health, University of Verona, Verona, Italy
*Corresponding author: e-mail address: dora.buonfrate@sacrocuore.it

Contents

† Contributed equally.

Advances in Parasitology, Volume 118
ISSN 0065-308X
https://doi.org/10.1016/bs.apar.2022.07.001

Abstract

Strongyloidiasis is the infection caused by soil-transmitted nematodes of *Strongyloides* species, infecting humans and some animals. *Strongyloides stercoralis* is the species with most clinical and epidemiological relevance in humans and dogs, due to its high prevalence and its capacity of inducing a life-threatening hyperinfection. Diagnosis of strongyloidiasis is challenging, due to the absence of a single reference standard test with high sensitivity and specificity, which also hampers the estimation of the accuracy of other diagnostic tests. In this chapter, we review the deployment and performance of the parasitological, immunological, molecular tests for the diagnosis of strongyloidiasis in humans and in dogs. Further, we comment the available evidence from genotyping studies that have addressed the zoonotic potential of *S. stercoralis*. Finally, we discuss the use of different diagnostic methods in relation to the purpose (i.e., screening, individual diagnosis, inclusion in a clinical trial) and the setting (endemic/non-endemic areas) and report the accuracy figures reported by systematic reviews on either parasitological, serological or molecular techniques published in literature.

1. Introduction

Strongyloidiasis is a parasitic infection caused by nematodes of the genus *Strongyloides*. An estimated 600 million people worldwide are infected by the species *S. stercoralis*, while rare human infections by *S. fuelleborni fuelleborni* have been reported in Africa and Asia (Bradbury et al., 2021b; Buonfrate et al., 2020). *S. fuelleborni kellyi* appears to be restricted to the island of New Guinea (Bradbury, 2021). Some *S. stercoralis* strains can also infect non-human primates, cats and dogs, posing concerns about a possible zoonotic transmission (Bradbury et al., 2021b; Gonzalez Akimori et al., 2021).

S. stercoralis is a soil-transmitted helminth: infection occurs by skin penetration of infective third-stage filariform larvae (iL3) living in the soil in areas with poor sanitation. The iL3 classically migrate through the blood vessels to the lungs, ascend the tracheobronchial tree and are swallowed into the intestinal tract, but they may also migrate directly through other tissues to the gastrointestinal tract (Page et al., 2018). During the migration route, they mature into different stages, and eventually settle in the wall of the small intestine as adult females (Nutman, 2017; Streit, 2008). The parasitic female reproduces by parthenogenesis, laying eggs that hatch into rhabditiform larvae (L1). In humans, these larvae are either excreted with faeces or transform into filariform larvae, which can penetrate the intestinal wall or the perianal skin, leading to reinfection. This is called 'auto-infective cycle', and causes the indefinite persistence of the infection, if left untreated (Nutman, 2017). When defecation occurs in the external environment, the L1 can either precociously develop into iL3 (direct or homogonic cycle) or into non-infective larvae, which go through different stages and eventually mature into free-living adult worms of both sexes (indirect or heterogonic cycle). The free-living adult worms reproduce sexually and their offspring moult twice to mature into iL3 (Streit, 2008). This second generation of the free-living cycle does not transform into adults and must find a host to complete the life cycle (Page et al., 2018).

As a result of the auto-infective cycle of *S. stercoralis* in humans, strongyloidiasis is a chronic infection. A large proportion of infected individuals present with no symptoms, while others present with intermittent, non-specific symptoms mostly affecting the skin and/or the gastrointestinal and/or the respiratory tracts (Buonfrate et al., 2021a). Eosinophilia may be intermittent or absent (Naidu et al., 2013), and this sign is frequent also in other parasitic infections, thus not specific (O'Connell and Nutman, 2016).

Immunosuppressed individuals can present with an accelerated autoinfective cycle, which leads to an increased larval load. This condition, named hyper-infection, usually manifests with worsening of symptoms and sometimes with sepsis by enteric bacteria, which can enter the bloodstream through intestinal ulceration (Nutman, 2017). In the most severe hyperinfection, there is a catastrophic dissemination of large numbers of larvae throughout body, with a high fatality rate (Buonfrate et al., 2013).

For chronic uncomplicated infection, first line treatment is ivermectin 200 μg/kg in a single dose, while albendazole demonstrates lower efficacy (Buonfrate et al., 2019; Henriquez-Camacho et al., 2016). Recent evidence suggests that moxidectin may become an alternative to the first line treatment (Hofmann et al., 2021). The treatment of infection in immunosuppressed individuals and hyperinfection relies on expert's opinion, and repeated doses of ivermectin are recommended up to 2 weeks from clearance from infection at microscopy examination of stool and/or previously-positive biological material (Nutman, 2017). In literature, hyperinfection cases treated with sub-cutaneous administration of ivermectin have been reported, some of them showing a good response to the treatment (Barrett et al., 2016).

S. f. fuelleborni is primarily a parasite of primates in Africa and Asia, but human infection is also rarely reported (Nutman, 2017). The disease resembles infection with *S. stercoralis*, though auto-infection seems unlikely since this species as eggs rather than larvae are passed (Pampiglione and Ricciardi, 1972; Potters et al., 2020). High intensity infections with *S. f. kellyi* due to external autoinfection rather than true autoinfection, has been associated with 'swollen belly syndrome', a severe protein-losing enteropathy in infants in New Guinea. In older ages, the prevalence and morbidity of this infection progressively reduces (Bradbury, 2021). There is scant evidence available about the best diagnostic and treatment approach for these subspecies.

The diagnosis of *S. stercoralis* infection is challenging, due to the intermittent shedding of larvae in the faeces and consequent low sensitivity of parasitological diagnosis. In addition, there is the absence of a single reference test with high sensitivity and specificity (Basáñez et al., 2004; Requena-Méndez et al., 2013). The lack of a single reference standard hampers a correct evaluation of novel diagnostic tests, the accuracy of which is often assessed against a panel of microscopy-positive samples, leading to over-estimation of the sensitivity and underestimation of the specificity of the novel test (Requena-Méndez et al., 2013). Alternative statistical methods have been recommended for the estimation of the accuracy of diagnostic tests in the absence of a single reference test (Rutjes et al., 2007), but these are still seldom applied. The application of different reference standards for the evaluation of accuracy sometimes hampers the comparison between diagnostic studies, thus this limitation should be taken into consideration also for meta-analyses.

Further, the choice of a diagnostic test should be based on the specific context and situation. Indeed, a diagnostic tool which is suitable for individual diagnosis in a non-endemic, high-income country, might not be so for use in screening surveys in endemic areas. The World Health Organization (WHO) has recently included the control of strongyloidiasis among the 2030 targets (Montresor et al., 2020), and the identification of a test that could be deployed in the field is compelling.

In this chapter, we review the tests for the diagnosis of strongyloidiasis in human and veterinary medicine, reporting assays used in routine practice for screening and diagnosis as well as experimental assays under evaluation/development.

2. Methods for literature search

2.1 Search strategy

We searched literature published from 1990 to November 6th 2021 and available in the following databases: MEDLINE, Google Scholar, Embase, Cochrane Central Register of Controlled Trials, LILACS. The complete list of keywords is reported in Table 1. Each author evaluated the record list generated by the search strategy and retrieved the papers to be included in the section he/she was in charge of. Further papers were retrieved from the reference list of included papers. Buonfrate and Tamarozzi also searched the records to retrieve systematic reviews on diagnostic methods for strongyloidiasis.

Table 1 Detailed search strategy used for literature search.

Database	Search terms
MEDLINE	(((((((((((((((("Strongyloides stercoralis"[Mesh]) OR "Strongyloides stercorali*"[Title/Abstract])) OR (("Strongyloidiasis"[Mesh]) OR ("Strongyloidiasis/diagnosis"[Mesh]) OR Strongyloidias*[Title/Abstract]))))))) OR (Anguillulias*[Title/Abstract])) OR (roundworm [Title/Abstract]))) AND ((((((("Serologic Tests"[Mesh:NoExp]) OR ("Sensitivity and Specificity"[Mesh]) OR Diagnos*[Title/Abstract])) OR ((Detect*[Title/Abstract] OR "diagnostic test"[Title/Abstract] OR assay*[Title/Abstract] OR immunoassays [Title/Abstract] OR "rapid test"[Title/Abstract]) OR ("Serological Tests"[Title/Abstract]

Continued

Table 1 Detailed search strategy used for literature search.—cont'd

Database	Search terms
	OR "Serological Test"[Title/Abstract] OR "Serologic Test"[Title/Abstract] OR Serodiagnos*[Title/Abstract] OR Microscopy[Title/Abstract] OR sedimentation[Title/Abstract] OR culture[Title/Abstract] OR "recombinant antigens"[Title/Abstract] OR antigen*[Title/Abstract]))) OR (Serodiagnosis[Title/Abstract] OR "Polymerase chain reaction (PCR)"[Title/Abstract] OR PCR[Title/Abstract] OR "Koga agar plate"[Title/Abstract] OR Koga[Title/Abstract] OR agar[Title/Abstract] OR Baermann[Title/Abstract] OR Kato-Katz[Title/Abstract] OR charcoal[Title/Abstract] OR "indirect fluorescent antibody test"[Title/Abstract] OR "IFAT"[Title/Abstract] OR "indirect fluorescent antibody"[Title/Abstract] AND "IFAT"[Title/Abstract] OR "indirect radioimmune antibody test (IRAT)[Title/Abstract])) OR ("enzyme-linked immunosorbent antibody assay (ELISA)"[Title/Abstract] OR ELISA (SsAg-ELISA)[Title/Abstract] OR "IgE-ELISAs"[Title/Abstract] OR "Bordier ELISA"[Title/Abstract] OR Immunoblot[Title/Abstract])) OR (("Western-Blot"[Title/Abstract] OR westernblot [Title/Abstract]))) OR ("immunochromatographic test (ICT)"[Title/Abstract] OR immunochromatographic[Title/Abstract] OR "ICT"[Title/Abstract] OR "luciferase immunoprecipitation system (LIPS)"[Title/Abstract] OR "luciferase immunoprecipitation system"[Title/Abstract] OR "LIPS"[Title/Abstract] OR "loop-mediated isothermal amplification (LAMP)"[Title/Abstract] OR "loop-mediated isothermal amplification"[Title/Abstract] OR "LAMP" [Title/Abstract] OR "Rapid IgG4 Lateral Flow Dipstick Test"[Title/Abstract])) OR ((IgG[Title/Abstract] OR IgG4[Title/Abstract] OR IgG1[Title/Abstract] OR IgE[Title/Abstract]) AND (antibod*[Title/Abstract])))
Embase	#1 'strongyloides stercoralis'/exp./mj OR 'strongyloidiasis'/exp./mj #2 'strongyloides stercoralis' OR 'strongyloidiasis' OR strongyloidias* OR anguillulias* OR roundworm:ti,ab #3 #1 OR #2 #4 'serology'/exp./mj OR 'sensitivity and specificity'/exp./mj #5 detect* OR 'diagnostic test' OR assay* OR immunoassays OR 'rapid test' OR 'serological tests' OR 'serological test' OR 'serologic test' OR serodiagnos* OR microscopy OR sedimentation OR culture OR 'recombinant antigens' OR antigen*:ti,ab #6 (serodiagnosis OR 'polymerase chain reaction (pcr)' OR pcr OR 'koga agar plate' OR koga OR agar OR baermann OR 'kato katz' OR charcoal OR 'indirect fluorescent antibody test' OR 'ifat' OR 'indirect fluorescent antibody ifat' OR 'indirect radioimmune

Table 1 Detailed search strategy used for literature search.—cont'd

Database	Search terms
	antibody test (irat)' OR 'enzyme-linked immunosorbent antibody assay (elisa)' OR elisa) AND 'ssag elisa' OR 'ige-elisas' OR 'bordier elisa' OR immunoblot OR 'western-blot' OR westernblot OR 'immunochromatographic test (ict)' OR immunochromatographic OR 'ict' OR 'luciferase immunoprecipitation system (lips)' OR 'luciferase immunoprecipitation system' OR 'lips' OR 'loop-mediated isothermal amplification (lamp)' OR 'loop-mediated isothermal amplification' OR 'lamp':ti,ab #7 'rapid igg4 lateral flow dipstick test' OR igg OR igg4 OR igg1 OR (ige NEAR/4 antibod*) #8 #4 OR #5 OR #6 OR #7 #9 #3 AND #8 #10 #9 AND [embase]/lim NOT ([embase]/lim AND [medline]/lim)
Cochrane	#1 MeSH descriptor: [Strongyloides stercoralis] explode all trees #2 MeSH descriptor: [Strongyloidiasis] explode all trees #3 (Strongyloides stercoralis OR Strongyloidias* OR Anguillulias* OR roundworm):ti,ab,kw #4 {OR #1-#3} #5 (Serodiagnosis OR 'Polymerase chain reaction (PCR)' OR PCR OR 'Koga agar plate' OR Koga OR agar OR Baermann OR Kato-Katz OR charcoal OR 'indirect fluorescent antibody test' OR 'IFAT' OR 'indirect fluorescent antibody IFAT' OR 'indirect radioimmune antibody test (IRAT)' OR 'enzyme-linked immunosorbent antibody assay (ELISA)' OR ELISA (SsAg-ELISA) OR 'IgE-ELISAs' OR 'Bordier ELISA' OR Immunoblot OR 'Western-Blot' OR westernblot OR 'immunochromatographic test (ICT)' OR immunochromatographic OR 'ICT' OR 'luciferase immunoprecipitation system (LIPS)' OR 'luciferase immunoprecipitation system' OR 'LIPS' OR 'loop-mediated isothermal amplification (LAMP)' OR 'loop-mediated isothermal amplification' OR 'LAMP' OR 'Rapid IgG4 Lateral Flow Dipstick Test' OR IgG OR IgG4 OR IgG1 OR IgE):ti,ab,kw #6 {AND #4-#5}
LILACS	(mj:(strongyloides stercoralis)) OR (mj:(strongyloidiasis)) AND (serological test) OR (diagnostic test) AND (db:("LILACS" OR "IBECS" OR "MedCarib" OR "CUMED" OR "LIPECS" OR "BINACIS" OR "SES-SP" OR "PAHOIRIS" OR "colecionaSUS" OR "BDENF"))

3. Results

The search retrieved 3663 records, which reduced to 3446 after duplicate removal. Eventually, 257 full-text papers were reviewed and quoted in this chapter. Three systematic reviews were identified and included here.

4. Coproparasitological methods

The peculiar life cycle of *S. stercoralis* means that larvae, not eggs, are eliminated with faeces. Furthermore, in chronic infections, the elimination of such larvae is scant and intermittent (Nutman, 2017). These two features are at the basis of the techniques used for the coproparasitological diagnosis of strongyloidiasis, and of their performances. Also, these features are responsible for the current absence of a reference standard for the diagnosis of infection to be used in clinical practice and research studies, since no single technique (coproparasitological, but also molecular and serological), at any given time, can achieve 100% sensitivity and specificity (Requena-Méndez et al., 2013).

Coproparasitological techniques classically used for the retrieval of helminth eggs and protozoan cysts, such as direct smear-based approaches (e.g. direct smear [DS], Kato-Katz [KK]), and gravity-based concentration techniques such as formalin-ether-based concentration techniques (FECT) and flotation techniques, have consistently lower sensitivity than methods developed for the specific retrieval of *S. stercoralis* larvae in faeces (Campo Polanco et al., 2014). These in turn basically exploit the capacity of the parasite larvae to migrate actively, variably combined with their capacity to enter the free-living life cycle, and are based on sedimentation (e.g. Baermann technique and its modifications), and culture (e.g. Agar Plate Culture [APC] and its modification). These techniques, although more sensitive, have several drawbacks that can impact on sensitivity in routine diagnostic use, including the need of fresh (ideally processed within a few hours from passing), unpreserved and unrefrigerated faeces. Concerning the latter, Ines et al. (Inês et al., 2011) compared the viability of *S. stercoralis* larvae using Baermann and APC when using fresh stool and stool stored at 4 °C for 24 h, 48 h and 72 h, and found that viability (and in parallel the sensitivity of the techniques) halved every 24 h of refrigeration. Furthermore, these techniques require longer times to obtain a result (up to 72 h or more for APC) and they carry the possible risk of infection for the operator manipulating samples possibly containing iL3. Finally, for all coproparasitological techniques requiring microscopic examination, knowledge that larvae of other parasites may be observed, and skills in differentiating them, are absolutely needed.

In general, it can be difficult to compare the accuracy of the different methods because of the huge variability in terms of setting, study design, reference test/combination of tests used, and actual specific protocol applied for each technique, including quantity of faeces processed and number of slides examined by microscopy at the end of the technique. Studies that made a dedicated comparison of these techniques are listed in Table 2. In the following paragraphs, we provide an overview of the techniques described in the literature and used in several settings for the diagnosis of strongyloidiasis, and their performances.

4.1 Direct smear and Kato-Katz techniques

The microscopic examination of faecal smears obtained by mixing a small quantity of stool with saline or iodine (direct smear technique [DS]) is probably the most widely used coproparasitological technique, especially in non-specialized centres, because of its simplicity and rapidity, although at the cost of very low sensitivity in the presence of light infections. This is understandable if one considers that only 2–5 mg of faeces are examined. For the diagnosis of strongyloidiasis, sensitivity is in the range of 0–18% (Campo Polanco et al., 2014; Chankongsin et al., 2020; de Kaminsky, 1993; Jongwutiwes et al., 1999; Koga et al., 1991; Lau Chong et al., 2005; Machicado et al., 2012; Meurs et al., 2017). Figures around 30–50% sensitivity were also reported (Getaneh et al., 2010; Hailegebriel et al., 2017; Hernández-Chavarría and Avendaño, 2001), but seem implausible.

The Kato-Katz (KK) technique is a semi-concentration method widely used for the quantitative assessment of eggs in faeces, especially in the context of epidemiological studies and control programs for the other soil-transmitted helminths (Cools et al., 2019). It was developed for the diagnosis of schistosomiasis in 1954 by Kato and Miura (Kato and Miura, 1954) and later adapted for field use by Katz and colleagues (Katz et al., 1972). The technique is not appropriate for the diagnosis of strongyloidiasis since it consistently fails to diagnose the infection (Carvalho et al., 2012; Lopez et al., 2016; Machicado et al., 2012; Schär et al., 2014).

4.2 Flotation techniques

Flotation techniques are based on the ability of parasite eggs and cysts to float on the surface of a solution (e.g. zinc sulphate) with higher density and adhere onto a glass slide placed on the solution meniscus surface

Table 2 Data summary from a selection studies comparing the diagnostic accuracy of different microscopic/coproculture assays for the detection of *Strongyloides stercoralis* from a single stool sample.

Location	**Honduras**	**Thailand**	**Thailand**	**Japan**	**Thailand**	**Brazil**	**Brazil**	**China**	**Ethiopia**	**Mozambique**	**Iran**
Reference	De Kaminsky (1993)	Jongwutiwes et al. (1999)	Koga et al. (1991)	Sato et al. (1995)	Sato et al. (1995)	Sato et al. (1995)	Blatt and Cantos (2003)	Steinmann et al. (2007)	Hailegebriel et al. (2017)	Meurs et al. (2017)	Mohammadi-Meskin et al. (2018)
Total specimens	427	1085	137	713	205	432	424	179	351	323	163
Positive by any method	70	191	31	109	98	49	23	21	43	100	27
(% positive)	**(16%)**	**(18%)**	**(23%)**	**(15%)**	**(48%)**	**(11%)**	**(5%)**	**(12%)**	**(12%)**	**(31%)**	**(17%)**
DS Positive	9	20	7	28	ND	ND	ND	ND	21	26	16
(%total positives)	**(13%)**	**(10%)**	**(23%)**	**(26%)**					**(49%)**	**(26%)**	**(59%)**
FEC Positive	ND	104	ND	44	54	13	16	ND	23	ND	8
(%total positives)		**(54%)**		**(40%)**	**(55%)**	**(26%)**	**(70%)**		**(53%)**		**(5%)**
Baermann	33	ND	ND	ND	ND	ND	16	9[a]	31	37	27
(%total positives)	**(47%)**						**(70%)**	**(43%)**	**(72%)**	**(37%)**	**(100%)**
H-M Positive	ND	93	18	30	ND	14	8	ND	19	70	26
(%total positives)		**(49%)**	**(58%)**	**(27%)**		**(29%)**	**(35%)**		**(44%)**	**(70%)**	**(96%)**

APC Positive	28[b]	186	30	105	95	46	23	13[c]	ND	83	22
(%total positives)	**(40%)**	**(97%)**	**(97%)**	**(96%)**	**(97%)**	**(94%)**	**(100%)**	**(62%)**		**(83%)**	**(81%)**
Charcoal culture	ND	ND	ND	ND	ND	ND	ND	ND	16	ND	ND
(%total positives)									**(37%)**		
Spontaneous sedimentation	ND	ND	ND	ND	ND	ND	14	ND	ND	ND	ND
(%total positives)							**(61%)**				

[a]18 (85.7% of total positives) detected when three stools tested.
[b]48 h—incubation only.
[c]21 (100% of total positives) detected when three stools tested.
ND = not done, APC: Agar plate culture, DS: Direct smear microscopy, FEC: Formalin-ether concentration, H-M: Harada-Mori culture.

(Faust et al., 1938; Willis, 1921). Flotation techniques have been assessed for the retrieval of *S. stercoralis* larvae, generally with poor results (sensitivity 4–8%) (Carvalho et al., 2012; Schär et al., 2014). Furthermore, the hyper-osmotic flotation solution rapidly distorts the larvae, making specific identification difficult. FLOTAC, and its modification Mini-FLOTAC, are flotation-based techniques for the quantitative diagnosis of faecal parasite elements (e.g. ova and cysts) using a 'closed' device (Cringoli et al., 2010, 2013). When evaluated for the diagnosis of strongyloidiasis by Glinz and colleagues (Glinz et al., 2010), their performance was poor, with only 2 positive samples detected of the 38 diagnosed by APC.

4.3 Sedimentation techniques

Protocols of faecal concentration based on the sedimentation of filtered, homogenized faeces have been applied since the early 1900s and have taken different names in the published literature (Faust et al., 1939; Hoffman et al., 1934; Lumbreras et al., 1962; Lutz, 1919). The Spontaneous in Tube Sedimentation Technique (STST), originally described by Tello and colleagues in 1988 (Tello et al., 2012), consists in the homogenization of faeces (about 10 g) with saline, followed by a spontaneous sedimentation step of the strained faeces in a 50 mL conical tube filled with saline or water. After at least 45 min, the sediment is examined by microscopy. The sedimentation can also be achieved by centrifugation (Inês et al., 2016). The Lumbreras rapid sedimentation test (Lumbreras et al., 1962), also widely used especially in Latin America, allows the homogenized and filtered faeces to settle for 45 min in a 200 mL conical vase filled with water. After discarding 2/3 of the supernatant, the vase is filled again and the sedimentation allowed for further 45 min. The sediment is then examined by microscopy, or the process repeated a few times before microscopy examination, until the supernatant is clear, depending on the protocol (Maco Flores et al., 2002). When applied for the diagnosis of strongyloidiasis, these sedimentation techniques were reported having sensitivity in the range of 27–75% (Blatt and Cantos, 2003; Carvalho et al., 2012; Hailu et al., 2021a; Inês et al., 2011; Lau Chong et al., 2005; Lopez et al., 2016; Machicado et al., 2012).

4.4 Formalin-ether concentration technique (FECT) and its modifications

FECT is a centrifugation-sedimentation method based on the different specific gravity of water and parasites (cysts, ova and larvae). Specifically, the parasites present in the formalin-fixed sample are heavier than the formalin-ether solution and settle in the sediment of the tube containing the mixture. In short, after centrifugation of homogenized faeces strained through gauze, four layers are formed, from the bottom: sediment, formalin, plug of lighter debris, and ether. Subsequent decanting of the supernatant and examination of the sediment by microscopy complete the process. The starting quantity of stool reported in the literature ranges from as much as an 'apricot-size' to as little as 500 mg.

The prototype of the FECT method was originally described by Telemann (Telemann, 1908) and modified by Ritchie (Ritchie, 1948), after whom the technique is commonly named. Several modifications of the 'Ritchie' technique have been described since, with slight changes in the quantity of faeces used and in the procedure steps (Allen and Ridley, 1970; Ridley and Hawgood, 1956). To overcome the disadvantages of the use of diethyl ether, which is flammable, explosive if exposed to light, and highly volatile with dispersion of anaesthetic vapour, several other chemicals have been evaluated as a substitute, first of all ethyl-acetate (Young et al., 1979). However, this chemical also is hazardous and several drawbacks in the processing of the sample and reading of the slide have been described (Erdman, 1981). Many further modifications of the FECT technique by use of different chemicals, less dangerous and/or more readily available, have been published, including gasoline (Ahmadi and Damraj, 2009), detergent (Anecimo et al., 2012; Kightlinger and Kightlinger, 1990), Tween (Ahmadi and Pakdad, 2007), D-Limonene (Hemo-De®) (Neimeister et al., 1987). Commercial devices for faecal examination using the FECT principle were also applied (Amor et al., 2016; Carvalho et al., 2012; Meurs et al., 2017; Perry et al., 1990). Generally speaking, all studies applying this vast array of modifications obtained similar results in respect to the (poorly sensitive) retrieval of *S. stercoralis* larvae. Reported sensitivity ranges from 6% to 60% (Anamnart et al., 2013; Arakaki et al., 1990; Aramendia et al., 2020; Blatt and Cantos, 2003; Carvalho et al., 2012; Getaneh et al., 2010; Hailegebriel et al., 2017; Intapan et al., 2005; Jongwutiwes et al., 1999; Kobayashi et al., 1996; Schär et al., 2014). In a systematic review and meta-analysis, Campo-Polanco and colleagues (Campo Polanco et al., 2014) estimated the global sensitivity of the FECT in 48% (95% CI 42–54%). Noteworthy, the reference standard of the reviewed studies were faecal-based techniques, only.

Anamnart et al. (Anamnart et al., 2010) evaluated the factors affecting the recovery rate of *S. stercoralis* by using FECT (2–4 g of known *S. stercoralis*-positive faeces), finding that the use of fresh faeces with only short time exposure to formalin (<2 h), use of a wire mesh instead of gauze, and a longer centrifugation time improved the recovery rate of larvae; however, sensitivity was increased only from 14% to 28% (Anamnart et al., 2010). By examining the other layers formed upon centrifugation, they found that a large proportion of larvae were actually trapped in the debris plug, in the gauze, and in the formalin layer (Anamnart et al., 2010). Furthermore, it has been argued that dead larvae are more difficult to discern in the sediment than moving larvae in a clear background as obtained by Baermann or culture techniques (Siddiqui and Berk, 2001). In a study that compared the microscopic detection of *Strongyloides* larvae in three stool specimens using direct smear, formalin ethyl acetate concentration and the solvent-free Parasep SF faecal concentrator (Apacor, Workingham, England), the Parasep SF concentrator was the least sensitive method (Moody et al., 2013).

4.5 Baermann funnel technique and its modifications

This technique was originally described in 1917 by the author naming it, who used it for the detection of hookworm larvae in soil, taking advantage of the thermotropism and hydrotrophism of larvae stimulating these to migrate spontaneously (Baermann, 1917), and later applied also to retrieve *S. stercoralis* larvae from faces (Coutinho et al., 1951; Moraers, 1948). The Baermann technique uses a specific apparatus consisting in a funnel fit with a short piece of tubing to the stem, closed at the other end by a clamp; the apparatus is supported by a stand or rack. Faeces (generally about 10 g) are placed in gauze and suspended in lukewarm water (30–45 °C) filling the apparatus, so that the sample only lightly touches the water. The active movement of larvae out of the faecal mass towards the water is allowed for a variable time at room temperature (generally between 25 °C and 30 °C), during which the larvae sediment at the lower extremity of the tube; sometimes a light is placed underneath the apparatus to further stimulate larval migration. Then, the last volume of water is transferred in a tube by loosening the clamp, centrifuged, and the sediment observed under the microscope. Several modifications have been applied to the original technique, for example, the use of a sedimentation flask instead of a funnel, with faeces partially (Lumbreras, 1959, 1963; Rugai et al., 1954) or completely (de Kaminsky, 1993) immersed in the lukewarm water; the use of laboratory tubes (Gelaye et al., 2021; Hernández Chavarria, 2001), or commercial kits (Willcox and Coura, 1989), or other materials more readily available in resource-poor settings, such as recycled plastic bottles (Graeff-Teixeira et al., 1997), with overall comparable results. Fig. 1 shows a Baermann apparatus.

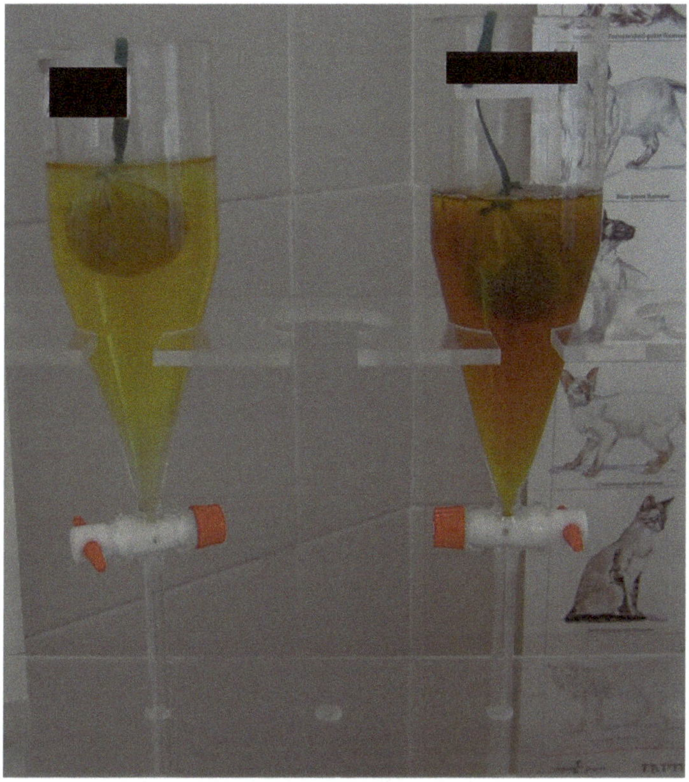

Fig. 1 Baermann apparatus with some modifications, since in this picture faeces are completely submerged in lukewarm water while in the classical technique faeces are suspended only lightly touching lukewarm water.

The technique has been also applied following APC culture (Inês et al., 2011) or coupled with a pre-incubation step with activated charcoal (Amor et al., 2016; Aramendia et al., 2020; Gelaye et al., 2021). Gelaye and colleagues (Gelaye et al., 2021), comparing three variations of the Baermann technique, found that the pre-incubation step of 3 g of stool with activated charcoal for 18–24 h at room temperature, followed by 2.5 h filtration through gauze, gave better results (sensitivity 87% when using results of all the three techniques combined as reference standard) than the same technique without pre-incubation (sensitivity 22.1%), and than the use of 10 g of stool pre-incubated with charcoal but allowed to filter through tissue paper for 1 h (sensitivity 26.7%). The authors (Gelaye et al., 2021) ascribed the better performance to the incubation procedure, which allowed the parasite to enter the free-living cycle, and the application of gauze instead of tissue paper in the filtration step, as well as the use of a smaller amount of faeces, both allowing larvae to move more freely towards the water.

Much variation in this technique is also described regarding the amount of faeces used, ranging from as much as >30 g (Amor et al., 2016; Aramendia et al., 2020; Salazar et al., 1995) to as little as 2 g (Gelaye et al., 2021), and in the filtration time, from 1 h to overnight (de Kaminsky, 1993; Gelaye et al., 2021; Graeff-Teixeira et al., 1997; Hailegebriel et al., 2017).

In published papers, the reported sensitivity of the Baermann technique ranges from 20% to 100% (Hernández-Chavarría and Avendaño, 2001; Knopp et al., 2008), most commonly, however, falling in the range of 40–80% (Aramendia et al., 2020; Becker et al., 2015; Blatt and Cantos, 2003; Carvalho et al., 2012; Chankongsin et al., 2020; de Kaminsky, 1993; Hailegebriel et al., 2017; Inês et al., 2011; Khieu et al., 2013; Krolewiecki et al., 2010; Lau Chong et al., 2005; Machicado et al., 2012; Meurs et al., 2017; Schär et al., 2014). In a systematic review and meta-analysis, Campo-Polanco and colleagues (Campo Polanco et al., 2014) estimated the global sensitivity of the Baermann technique at 72% (95% CI 67–76%).

4.6 Agar plate culture (APC) and its modifications

The use of agar plate to culture *S. stercoralis* was first described by Arakaki and colleagues in 1988, developed from the observation that occasionally bacterial colonies grew in the form of furrows in coprocultures using nutrient agar plates for bacteriology (Arakaki et al., 1988). The APC technique takes advantage of the capacity of the parasite to develop its free-living cycle, and the method was standardized by Koga and colleagues (Koga et al., 1991). Briefly, about 2–3 g of stool are placed at the centre of a nutrient 1.5% agar sterile medium (containing 0.5% meat extract, 1% peptone and 0.5% NaCl) in a Petri dish and incubated at room temperature (26–33 °C). Cultures are maintained generally for 48 h, although prolongation until 7 days may increase the detection rate (Jongwutiwes et al., 1999). Tracks resulting from bacterial growth along the path of larval movement may not be always macroscopically evident, or even visible after examination of the plate by microscopy; therefore, careful washing of the plate surface using 10% formalin or water and observation of the sediment by microscopy are required to complete the reading (Koga et al., 1991).

In their original study, Arakaki and colleagues (Arakaki et al., 1988) found that using a 37 °C incubation of finger-head size stool for 48 h, *S. stercoralis* could be detected in 4.5–5.7% samples from patients accessing their clinic, compared to 0% by DS, 0.3% by Harada-Mori test tube culture, and 0.8% by FECT. Based on results from cultures with serial dilution of faeces containing a known number of larvae, Koga and colleagues (Koga et al., 1992) estimated that at least 3 g of stool should be used. Optimal culture conditions were further described by Kaewrat and colleagues (Kaewrat et al., 2020) and confirmed by Senthong and colleagues (Sengthong et al., 2020), using a yeast extract-based agar with 0.5% NaCl, pH 6.0 and incubation temperature of 29–30 °C. However, also non-nutrient agar using 1% plain food agar has been tested and reported similar performance to nutrient agar (Sukhavat et al., 1994). A recent study in Thailand found that use of Oxoid™ nutrient agar adjusted to pH 6.0 was superior to the Koga agar formulation for the recovery of larvae (Kaewrat et al., 2020).

To prevent larvae from crawling out of the plate, with consequent alteration of results and risk of infection for the operator, Arakaki et al. (Arakaki et al., 1988) suggested the use of a double-walled Petri dish with 25% glycerine half-filling the outer space between the plates (Arakaki et al., 1990). This has been replaced by simply sealing the Petri dish using sealing films (Koga et al., 1991).

A modification of the APC technique was described by Khanna and colleagues (Khanna et al., 2015), which requires the cutting of a 1 cm wide canal around a square area of 2 × 2 cm in an agar plate, which is then filled with saline or water. About 2 g of stool are placed on the central square area and incubated for 3 days; larvae and adults could then be retrieved from the liquid in the canal using a pipette introduced through a hole in the plate lid, without the need to open the plate and wash the surface of the agar. While the authors declared that this technique 'had better yield of parasites' compared to the conventional APC method (Khanna et al., 2015), no actual figures were provided.

APC is generally considered the most sensitive coproparasitological technique for the diagnosis of *S. stercoralis* infection, with reported sensitivity in the range of 60–98% (Arakaki et al., 1990; Blatt and Cantos, 2003; Chankongsin et al., 2020; Hailegebriel et al., 2017; Hailu et al., 2021b; Hernández-Chavarría and Avendaño, 2001; Inês et al., 2011; Intapan et al., 2005; Jongwutiwes et al., 1999; Khieu et al., 2013; Kobayashi et al., 1996; Koga et al., 1991; Lau Chong et al., 2005; Machicado et al., 2012; Schär et al., 2014) although lower figures (20–50%) are also reported (Anamnart et al., 2013; Becker et al., 2015; Buonfrate et al., 2017b; de Kaminsky, 1993; Knopp et al., 2008; Krolewiecki et al., 2010). In a systematic review and meta-analysis, Campo-Polanco and colleagues (Campo Polanco et al., 2014) estimated the global sensitivity of the APC technique in 89% (95% CI 86–92%).

4.7 Filter paper-based culture techniques

The Harada-Mori technique was described in 1955 for the diagnosis of hookworm by the authors after whom it is named (Harada and Mori, 1955). Around 1 g of fresh faeces are smeared on a 2–3 cm wide filter paper strip. One of the clear extremities of the strip is dipped into water contained in a tube and incubated at 20–30 °C for 3–10 days. The water is then centrifuged and the sediment examined under the microscope for the presence of larvae.

Another filter paper-based culture technique consists in mixing equal parts of fresh stool and activated charcoal or vermiculite in the centre of a Petri dish layered with moisten filter paper, incubated for several days while maintaining the moisture; larvae are retrieved from the plate by further addition of water at the end of the incubation period, and observed under a microscope (Hailegebriel et al., 2017; Meurs et al., 2017; Polderman et al., 2010).

These methods have generally lower sensitivities (in the range of 19–57%) compared to the APC and Baermann techniques (Blatt and Cantos, 2003; Hailegebriel et al., 2017; Jongwutiwes et al., 1999; Kobayashi et al., 1996; Koga et al., 1991; Krolewiecki et al., 2010; Machicado et al., 2012; Meurs et al., 2017).

4.8 Other reported techniques based on larval migration

A number of other techniques taking advantage of larval migration have been described. Dancescu (Dancescu, 1968) described a method consisting in mixing equal parts of charcoal and faeces (6–9 g each) in a cone-shape inside a small box of transparent plastic, with the top of the cone touching the inner surface of the transparent lid of the box. After incubation, larvae can be observed in the condensation drops through microscopic observation of the inner surface of the lid. Lau-Chong and colleagues (Lau Chong et al., 2005) applied this technique in a field study in Peru, finding a sensitivity of 92.3% when the reference standard was positivity in any of the applied DS, STST, Baermann in flask, and APC.

The water-emergence technique consists in producing a central depression in a fresh stool specimen, filled with lukewarm water, and incubated at 37 °C for 1 h to allow larvae to migrate into the dip. These can be then recovered and examined by microscopy. In their study in the hospital setting in Ethiopia, Gataneh and colleagues (Getaneh et al., 2010) found that this technique had a sensitivity of 85.1% when the reference standard was positivity in any of the applied DS, FECT and water-emergence tests.

4.9 Strategies to improve detection rates by coproparasitological techniques

Different coproparasitological techniques can be applied on the same sample to achieve better sensitivity since it is a common finding that there is imperfect or even limited overlap between samples found positive with one or with another result from different methods in an examined population (Anamnart et al., 2013; Aramendia et al., 2020; Becker et al., 2015; de Kaminsky, 1993; Inês et al., 2011; Intapan et al., 2005; Kobayashi et al., 1996). The same applies when molecular techniques (PCR on stool) are performed in parallel to coproparasitological techniques such as APC or Baermann (Amor et al., 2016; Aramendia et al., 2020; Becker et al., 2015; Buonfrate et al., 2017b; Chankongsin et al., 2020; Kristanti et al., 2018; Krolewiecki et al., 2010; Meurs et al., 2017; Schär et al., 2013).

To deal with the problem of intermittent elimination of larvae and of the low number of larvae generally eliminated in chronic infections, the diagnostic sensitivity could also be increased by increasing the amount of faeces examined, and examining multiple samples produced in different days by the same individual (Dacal et al., 2018; Dreyer et al., 1996; Khieu et al., 2013; Knopp et al., 2008; Lopez et al., 2016; Nielsen and Mojon, 1987; Repetto et al., 2016; Sato et al., 1995; Steinmann et al., 2007; Uparanukraw et al., 1999). However, infection confirmation proves generally difficult. Sato and colleagues (Sato et al., 1995) applied multiple coproparasitological techniques (DS, FECT, and APC) to re-confirm *S. stercoralis* infection 5 and 18 months after initial diagnosis and found that maximum rate of reconfirmation was achieved by APC. However, this reconfirmation rate was unsatisfactory, with only 60% of infections re-detected by APC when performed once, and 85% when re-performed on three specimens collected on different days. Re-detection rates by other techniques ranged from 16% (DS)—24% (FECT) when performed on one stool specimen, to 45% (FECT)—51% (DS) when performed on three specimens (Sato et al., 1995). Uparanukraw and colleagues (Uparanukraw et al., 1999) found that 9.8% of individuals initially deemed negative based on a single APC-negative result were actually infected when up to 6 consecutive specimens over a month were cultured; furthermore, up to 8 consecutive examinations by APC over 2 months were necessary to re-confirm all 56 *S. stercoralis*-positive individuals initially diagnosed as infected in their cohort. Dreyer et al. (Dreyer et al., 1996) applied the Baermann-Moraes technique weekly over 2 months using 25 g of faeces and examining the whole sediment of 40 mL sedimentation fluid (about 100 slides/sample) in 108 patients with proven *S. stercoralis* infection, finding that the maximum sensitivity ($n=72$; 66.7%) for the scheduled timeframe was achieved at the 4th weekly examination. The remaining 36 patients had a positive Baermann only between week 9 and 21, always with weekly examinations. Furthermore, elimination was not constant week to week in individual patients, although those with detectable larvae over consecutive weeks tended to eliminate larvae more constantly over time than the others. Single specimen examination had a sensitivity ranging from 19.4% to 36.1% (Dreyer et al., 1996). In a study conducted in Tanzania, it was estimated that up to 12 samples collected in different days would have to be analysed by APC and up to 20 by Baermann if $\leq$1% false negative results were allowed (Knopp et al., 2008). Similarly, when using the mathematical model developed by Marti and Koella (Marti and Koella, 1993) to estimate the "true" prevalence of helminth infection based on examination of multiple stool samples, Steinmann and colleagues in China (Steinmann et al., 2007) found that sensitivity of single APC or single Baermann were 63% and 48%, respectively, while increased to 95% and 86%, respectively, when three stool samples collected on consecutive days were examined; using APC with three samples, the estimated *S. stercoralis* prevalence in the investigated province (11.7%) reached the 'true' prevalence calculated by the mathematical model (12.3% $\pm$ 5.1%).

4.10 Identification of *S. stercoralis* in diagnostic preparations and differential diagnosis with other parasites

Already during the first studies using the APC (Arakaki et al., 1990), the emergence of larvae of different species was observed, especially after 48 h incubation, flagging the importance of differentiating the retrieved parasites (Arakaki et al., 1990; Inês et al., 2011; Jongwutiwes et al., 1999; Koga et al., 1991). The same applies in case of delayed processing from the time of defecation.

The shape of tracks on agar and the movement pattern of the larvae could be of some use in their identification, but these parameters cannot be completely relied upon, and careful morphological identification is always required (Inês et al., 2011; Jongwutiwes et al., 1999). Furthermore, tracks are not always visible in positive samples; therefore, it is important to carry out microscopic examination of the surface and of the plate surface washing sediment also of plates with no visible furrows (de Kaminsky, 1993). Depending on the time elapsing from stool production to microscopic examination of the processed sample, several stages of *S. stercoralis* can be observed, which should be differentiated from larvae of other parasites hatching from eggs upon culture, depending on areas of co-endemicity (Blotkamp et al., 1993; Bradbury, 2019, 2021; Grove, 1996).

L1 (Fig. 2) are 180–240 μm long, with a shallow buccal capsule and a muscular oesophagus which occupies the anterior one-third of the body, divided into an anterior cylindrical corpus and a posterior rounded bulb. L1 can be observed within 1–2 days in freshly passed stool or after culture, produced by free-living adult worms (Figs. 3 and 4) developed in cultured faecal samples. *S. stercoralis* L1 can be differentiated from hookworm, *Trichostrongylus* spp., *Oesophagostomum* spp., *Ternidens deminutus* and *Rhabditis* spp. L1 mainly on the basis of the short buccal capsule and prominent rhomboid genital primordium placed about half-way down the length of the larva (Fig. 5). L1 of *T. deminutus* also have prominent, though smaller, genital primordium. However, these may easily be differentiated from L1 *S. stercoralis* by their larger size (300–360 μm), longer buccal cavities and long flagella-like tails.

Through an L2 stage, characterized by a progressive lengthening of the body and of the oesophagus, iL3 develop after further 1–2 days of culture (Fig. 6). *S. stercoralis* filariform larvae are 490–630 μm long and slender, with a typical filariform oesophagus, and are characterized by a notched tail and a 1:1 oesophagus to intestine ratio (Fig. 6). Fig. 7 shows the morphology of filariform larvae of different helminths.

Hatched larvae of *S. f. fuelleborni* and of S. *f. kellyi* are indistinguishable from those of *S. stercoralis*; these species can be differentiated in their cultured free-living adult stages, although morphological differences are subtle (Speare, 1989).

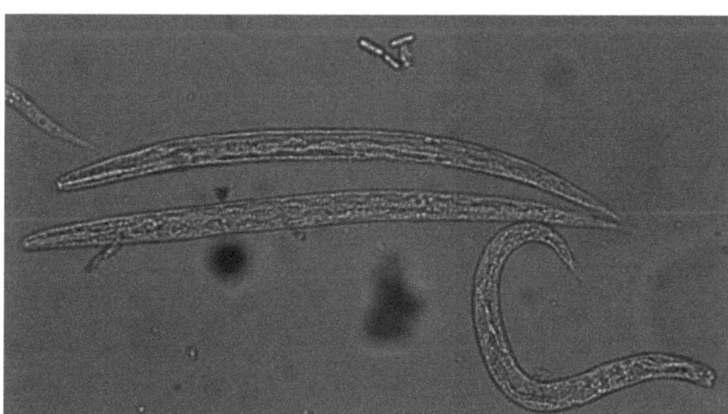

Fig. 2 *S. stercoralis* rhabditiform (L1) larvae from Baermann sedimentation. Note the shallow buccal cavity characterizing this stage in this species.

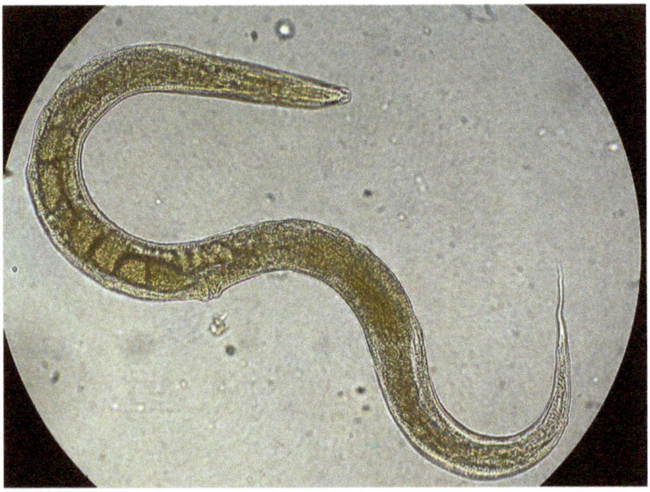

Fig. 3 *S. stercoralis* adult female from APC culture. The axis of the vulva perpendicular to the longitudinal axis of the parasite and the absence of body diameter narrowing after the vulvar opening are characteristics of *S. stercoralis* free-living adult females.

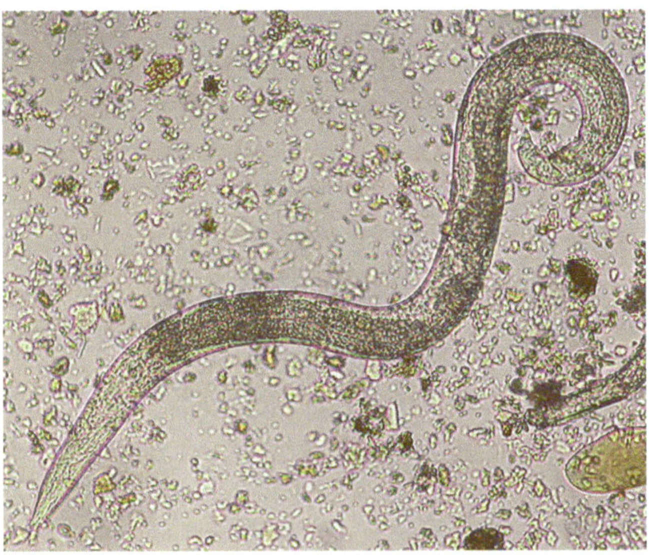

Fig. 4 *S. stercoralis* adult male from APC culture. The shape of the spiculae, visible towards the posterior end of the parasite, can be used for *Strongyloides* species identification.

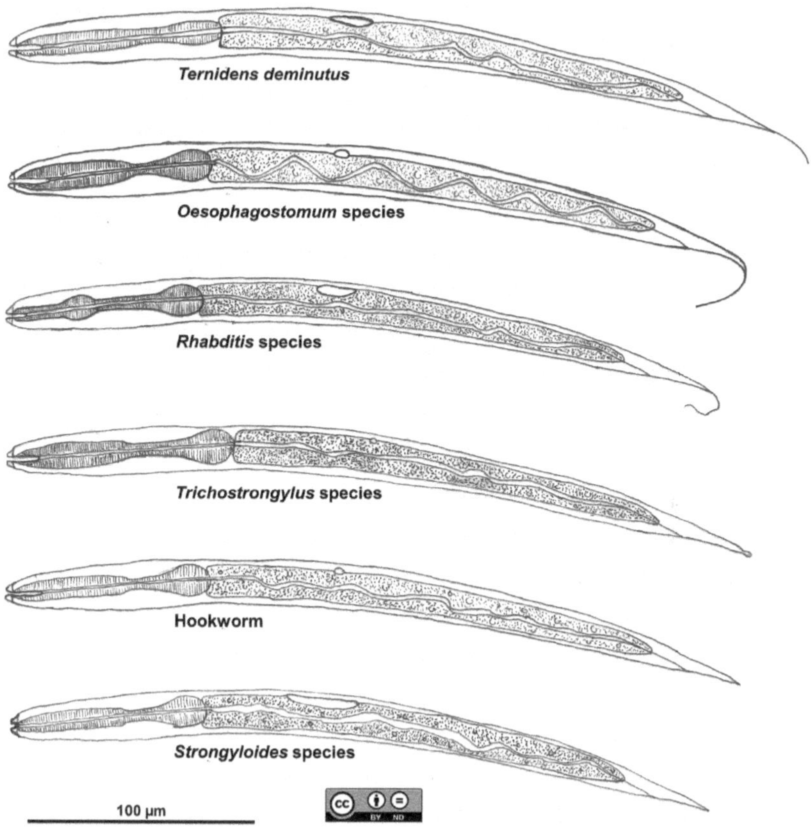

Fig. 5 Morphological comparison of rhabditiform (L1) larvae which may be cultured from human faeces. *Note*: The L1 and L2 rhabditiform larvae of the human hookworms (*Ancylostoma ceylanicum, Ancylostoma duodenale* and *Necator americanus*) are morphologically indistinguishable. The whip-like tail of *Oesophogostomum* species is longer than shown here when compared to total body length in the L2 stage. All larvae have extended body lengths, particularly in the intestinal region, in the L2 stage*. * *Image permission by Richard Bradbury.*

Unfortunately, little attention is given today to the maintenance of 'classic' parasitology skills, including morphology, in the curriculum of health-care professional figures who may be involved in various aspects of diagnostic parasitology. This often leads to incorrect species identification, adding to the problems in accurate mapping of infection and evaluation of diagnostic techniques and treatment interventions inherent in the biology of the parasite.

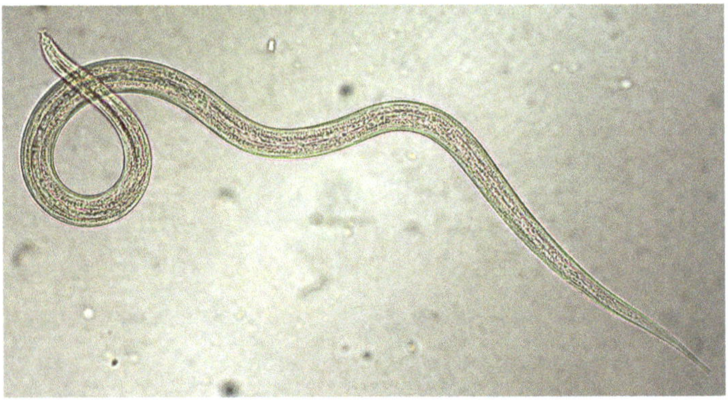

Fig. 6 *S. stercoralis* filariform (L3) larva. Note the notched tail characterizing this species stage.

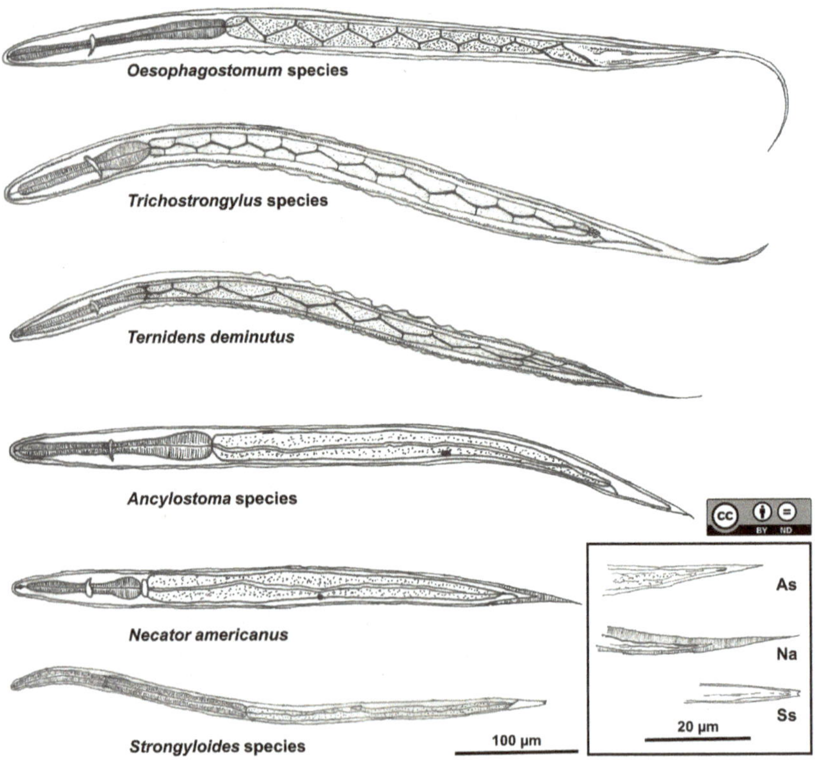

Fig. 7 Morphological comparison of filariform (L3) larvae which may be cultured from human faeces. (Inset): comparison of tail morphology of *Ancylostoma* species (As), *Necator americanus* (Na) and *Strongyloides* species (Ss). *Note*: Although various *Rhabditis* species have been reported from human faeces, to the best of the author's knowledge, none of these reports have described the morphology of the L3 larvae at the time of writing*. * *Image permission by Richard Bradbury.*

5. Immunodiagnosis

5.1 Serodiagnosis with enzyme-linked immunosorbent assays (ELISAs)

The use of tests based on antibody detection have been widely adopted in non-endemic countries for the screening of strongyloidiasis. This is mostly due to the availability of commercial enzyme-linked immunosorbent assays (ELISAs), which are easy to perform and less time-consuming compared to parasitological methods. In addition, several in-house assays have been described in the literature. Overall, the accuracy reported is good, though differences in the reference standard and panel of samples used to estimate sensitivity and specificity prohibit comparative evaluation of the performance of individual tests. The ELISAs maybe differentiated into assays based on crude antigens retrieved from *Strongyloides* larvae and those using recombinant antigens, as specified in the following paragraphs. Table 3 reports the sensitivity and specificity values of different ELISAs, as estimated in selected diagnostic studies. We included in the table only studies comparing at least two different assays and reporting confidence intervals.

5.1.1 Crude antigen-based ELISAs

ELISAs commercially available at the time of writing detect IgG-class antibodies to crude antigens (CrAg) extracted from different species of *Strongyloides,* including *S. stercoralis*, *S. ratti*, and *S. papillosus* (Bon et al., 2010; Buonfrate et al., 2021b; van Doorn et al., 2007). The use of antigens from species not infecting humans is due to the risk of infectivity with *S. stercoralis* for the laboratory staff and to an easier access to antigen sources, due to the possibility of maintaining the life cycle of the parasites in the laboratory (Huaman et al., 2003; Nutman, 2017; Sykes and McCarthy, 2011).

Overall, the high sensitivity, ranging from 83% to 95% (Bisoffi et al., 2014; Bon et al., 2010; Buonfrate et al., 2021b; Fradejas et al., 2018; Ruantip et al., 2019; van Doorn et al., 2007) is the main strength of the CrAg ELISAs available on the market. Specificity, ranging from 42.1% to 97.4% (Bisoffi et al., 2014; Bon et al., 2010; Buonfrate et al., 2021b; Fradejas et al., 2018; Ruantip et al., 2019; van Doorn et al., 2007) is influenced by possible cross-reactions with other helminths, such as filarial nematodes and *Schistosoma* spp. (Bisoffi et al., 2014; van Doorn et al., 2007). Although the result provided in routine practice is qualitative, increasing levels of the normalised optical density (nOD), which is the signal to cut-off ratio, were associated to higher specificity in diagnostic studies (Bisoffi et al., 2014).

Table 3 Selection of studies reporting the diagnostic accuracy of different serology assays.

		Crude Antigen ELISAs			Recombinant antigen ELISAs				Other assays	
Study	**Reference standard**	**ELISA SciMedx Denville, NJ, US**	**ELISA Microwell IVD Research, Inc., Carlsbad, CA, US**	**ELISA Bordier Affinity Products SA, Crissier, Switzerland**	**NIE ELISA NovaTec Immuno-diagnostica, Dietzenbach, Germany**	**NIE ELISA InBios Int, Inc., Seattle, WA, US**	**NIE ELISA by the National Institute of Health, Bethesda, Maryland, US**	**NIE-SsIR ELISA InBios Int, Inc., Seattle, WA, US**	**NIE LIPS by the National Institute of Health, Bethesda, Maryland, US**	**IFAT (in-house technique from IRCCS Sacro Cuore Don Calabria, Negrar, Verona, Italy)**
Bisoffi et al., 2014	Parasitological tests (including FECT, Baermann and APC)		Sens 91.2% (95% CI 86.0–96.4%) Spec 91.9% (95% CI 88.8–95.1%)	Sens 89.5% (95% CI 83.8–95.1) Spec 88.8% (95% CI 85.1–92.4%)			Sens 75.4% (95% CI 67.5–83.3%) Spec 89.5% (95% CI 85.9–93.0%)		Sens 85.1% (95% CI 78.5–91.6%) Spec 95.4% (95% CI 93.0–97.9%)	Sens 93.9% (95% CI 89.4–98.3%) Spec 82.5% (95% CI 78.0–86.9%)
	Composite reference standard (including the above-mentioned tests and serology)		Sens 92.3% (95% CI 87.8–96.9%) Spec 97.4% (95% CI 95.5–99.3%)	Sens 90.8% (95% CI 85.8–95.7%) Spec 94.0% (95% CI 91.2–96.9%)			Sens 70.8% (95% CI 62.9–78.6%) Spec 91.1% (95% CI 87.7–94.5%)		Sens 83.8% (95% CI 77.5–90.2%) Spec 99.6% (95% CI 98.9–100.0%)	Sens 94.6% (95% CI 90.7–98.5%) Spec 87.4% (95% CI 83.4–91.3%)
Fradejas et al., 2018	Parasitological tests (including FECT, APC) and PCR)	Sens 94.7% (95% CI 75.4–99%) Spec 72.3% (95% CI 58.2–83.1%)			Sens 78.9% (95% CI 56.7–91.5%) Spec 85.1% (95% CI 72.3–92.6%)					

	Composite reference standard (including the above-mentioned tests, serology and epidemiological risk factors)	Sens 89.2% (95% CI 80.7–94.2%) Spec 89.3% (95% CI 83.1–93.4%)	Sens 72.3% (95% CI 81.8–80.8%) Spec 85.1% (95% CI 72.3–92.6%)		
Ruantip et al., 2019	Parasitological methods (including APC and FECT)	Sens 91% (95% CI 75.8–97.8) Spec 42.1% (95% CI 21.1–66.0%)		Sens 82.9% (95% CI 65.7–92.8%) Spec 57.9% (95% CI 40.0–78.9%)	
Tamarozzi et al., 2021	Parasitological tests (including FECT, APC) and PCR)				Sens of IgG 93% (95% CI 88–97%) Spec of IgG 91% (95% CI 88–95%) Sens of IgG4 81% (95% CI 74–87%) Spec of IgG4 94% (95% CI 91–97%)
	Composite reference standard (including the above-mentioned tests and serology)				Sens of IgG 76% (95% CI 71–82%) Spec of IgG 98% (95% CI 96–100%) Sens of IgG4 75% (95% CI 69–81) Spec of IgG4 91% (95% CI 88–95%)

A commercial CrAg ELISA demonstrated excellent agreement of results obtained from serum compared to those obtained from dried blood spots collected on filter paper (Formenti et al., 2016; Tilli et al., 2021). This would be useful for fieldwork, as transport and storage of samples from remote areas would be easier.

In literature, different in-house CrAg ELISAs have also been evaluated, with sensitivity and specificity ranges similar to those observed for the commercial assays (Brasil et al., 1988; Eamudomkarn et al., 2015; Lindo et al., 1993; Loutfy et al., 2002; Machado et al., 2003; Ruantip et al., 2019; Sithithaworn et al., 2003; van Doorn et al., 2007).

Seroreversion usually occurs after treatment, although it requires several months (Biggs et al., 2009; Buonfrate et al., 2015; Loutfy et al., 2002; Page et al., 2006; Kearns et al., 2017). Thus, false positive cases due to previous infections are presumably limited to recently treated cases. The seroreversion allows using these tests to monitor the response to treatment and, in case of quantitative result, a decrease of the nOD can be gradually observed over time (Buonfrate et al., 2015).

Drawbacks of the CrAg ELISAs are the lower specificity compared to parasitological methods, variable reproducibility between different batches of the assays, due to different antigen lots, and the difficulties related to the production of filariform larvae for antigen extraction, which is time-consuming and hampers the production of large quantities of the assay (Pak et al., 2014). Moreover, sensitivity might be lower in immunosuppressed individuals, with a reduced antibody response (Abdul-Fattah et al., 1995; Ahmed et al., 2019) and in very early infection (Ming et al., 2019).

5.1.2 Recombinant antigen-based ELISAs

In order to overcome these issues, ELISAs based on recombinant antigens have been implemented, most of them currently available for research-use-only (RUO). The recombinant antigens most frequently used are a 31-kDa antigen derived from the L3 cDNA library, named NIE (Ravi et al., 2002), and the *S. stercoralis* immunoreactive antigen, SsIR (Ramanathan et al., 2008). The sensitivity and specificity of ELISAs based on NIE range between 70.8–97% and 57.9–95% (Anderson et al., 2014; Bisoffi et al., 2014; Fradejas et al., 2018; Ramanathan et al., 2008; Ruantip et al., 2019), respectively. Similar to what observed for CrAg ELISAs, a RUO NIE ELISA proved useful for post-treatment monitoring, both at individual and at community level (Buonfrate et al., 2015; Ramanathan et al., 2008; Vargas et al., 2017). Further, the same test demonstrated excellent agreement between results obtained on serum with those obtained from dried blood spots (Mounsey et al., 2014). More recently, ELISAs using a combination of NIE and SsIR have been implemented, to further improve the accuracy of the tests. A novel NIE/SsIR assay detecting IgG demonstrated good performance in a retrospective diagnostic study (Tamarozzi et al., 2021), with 78% sensitivity (95% CI: 72–83%) and 98% specificity (95% CI: 96–100%). In the same study, a NIE/SsIR ELISA detecting IgG4 showed lower accuracy, with sensitivity and specificity of 70% (64–76) and 97% (95–100), respectively.

5.1.3 Other experimental ELISAs

Some experimental ELISAs detecting different immunoglobulin isotypes and subclasses (such as IgG1, IgG4, IgE and IgA) (Ahmad et al., 2020; Arifin et al., 2013; Atkins et al., 1997; Norsyahida et al., 2013; Rodrigues et al., 2007) have been evaluated, with the aim of improving the specificity of the assay and/or the capacity of diagnosing acute infection. In particular, IgG4 is the subclass most studied, deemed promising for the high specificity for helminth intestinal infections (Arifin et al., 2019; Norsyahida et al., 2013). However, the results are still inconsistent, and the reduced sensitivity of these assays compared to IgG-based ELISAs, in particular during chronic infection (such as IgG1 and IgE which are probably downregulated during chronic infection) (Ahmad et al., 2020; Arifin et al., 2013; Atkins et al., 1997; Kubofcik and Nutman, 2016; Ramanathan et al., 2008) has so far limited their implementation.

In the last decade, the Phage Display technology has been deployed to identify peptides mimicking *S. stercoralis* antigens (mimotopes), which can be used for the implementation of phage ELISAs (Levenhagen et al., 2021). Phage-based tests would have the advantages of high reproducibility, low cost and potential massive production (Feliciano et al., 2014; Levenhagen et al., 2021; Miguel et al., 2020). Moreover, the Phage Display technology has been used to select functional probes that can detect immune complexes circulating in *S. stercoralis* infected individuals. Tests based on these probes would have the advantage of identifying active infection (Levenhagen et al., 2021; Miguel et al., 2020).

Also, the use of biological materials other than blood/serum has been evaluated, in order to make sample collection more accessible and accepted by individuals. An in-house ELISA to detect IgG in urine had fair agreement ($k=0.615$) with the results of the same assay using serum (Ruantip et al., 2019). Other authors found either IgG, IgA or IgG immune complexes in saliva, using in-house ELISAs (Bosqui et al., 2015, 2017). These techniques still need further evaluation of their accuracy.

5.2 Other assays based on antibody detection

Among the different assays that have been evaluated for the detection of *S. stercoralis* antibodies, the luciferase immunoprecipitation system (LIPS) is probably the one that demonstrated the best performance so far, in particular in terms of specificity, compared to CrAg and recombinant antigen ELISAs (Bisoffi et al., 2014; Krolewiecki et al., 2010; Ramanathan et al., 2008). The test is based on the fusion of a specific antigen with the enzyme reporter *Renilla* luciferase (Ruc). A mixture of Ruc and patient serum is transferred to a plate containing A/G beads which capture IgG molecules. The antibody bound Ruc-antigen is then visualized by luminometer (Ramanathan et al., 2008). LIPS is a technology which allows obtaining a quantification of antigen-specific antibodies in a relatively short time. Compared to ELISAs, the background noise is extremely reduced, leading to a high signal (Ramanathan et al., 2008). LIPS assays based on either NIE or the combination of NIE and SsIR were evaluated for the detection of IgG and IgG4 to *S. stercoralis*. Overall, sensitivity and specificity ranged from 87% to 100% and from 91% to 100%, with the lowest sensitivity values estimated in the IgG4 format (Bisoffi et al., 2014; Krolewiecki et al., 2010; Ramanathan et al., 2008). Despite the excellent performance, this assay is not widely available, and the ELISA format is still considered a more practical solution for routine use.

Other in-house techniques that have been described in the literature include immunofluorescence tests (IFAT) and immunoblot techniques (Andreetta Corral et al., 2019; Bisoffi et al., 2014; Boscolo et al., 2007; Conway et al., 1993; Lindo et al., 1993; Machado et al., 2008). Immunoblots have also been used to identify other potential biomarkers (Sudré et al., 2007; Varatharajalu et al., 2011; Corral et al., 2015; Andreetta Corral et al., 2019). The assays differ widely between each other for the target proteins. Overall, the sensitivity and specificity of the assays range between 82–97% and 96–100% (Lindo et al., 1993; Silva et al., 2003; Machado et al., 2008), respectively. A biplex Western blot based on the recombinant antigens NIE and SsRI detecting IgG4 was implemented recently, showing high sensitivity and specificity in an experimental study (de Souza et al., 2021). IFAT assays have been implemented using antigens from either *S. stercoralis* or different species; overall, they demonstrated good sensitivity and specificity, ranging from 87%–95% and 87%–100%, respectively (Boscolo et al., 2007; Bisoffi et al., 2014; Buonfrate et al., 2017b; Costa-Cruz et al., 1997; Koosha et al., 2004; Silva et al., 2003; Gottardi et al., 2015). The test proved also useful for post-treatment monitoring

(Buonfrate et al., 2015; Boscolo et al., 2007). Although accuracy proved similar or slightly better than ELISA assays, they have a more laborious execution and interpretation, so they are less deployed in routine practice.

Other assays were implemented with the aim of developing rapid, easy-to-use tests, which could also be deployed in remote endemic areas. These are the gelatin particle agglutination tests (GPAT) and the immunochromatographic tests (ICT). Experimental GPAT were implemented through sensitization of gelatin particles with either *S. stercoralis* or other species (Ahmed et al., 2019; Huaman et al., 2003; Sithithaworn et al., 2005). They demonstrated good accuracy, with increased sensitivity compared to ELISAs, in particular for diagnosis in immunocompromised individuals (Ahmed et al., 2019; Huaman et al., 2003). However, the number of published studies is still limited for a thorough evaluation of this technique.

ICT, or lateral-flow assays, are easy-to-use and rapid point-of-care tests. Some prototypes based on *S. stercoralis* CrAg showed good sensitivity (ranging from 91% to 93.3%) and specificity (from 83.7% to 97.7%) (van Doorn et al., 2007; Sadaow et al., 2020). To overcome the same limitations listed for the CrAg—ELISAs, ICT based on recombinant antigens were also implemented. A dipstick test detecting IgG4 and based on the combination of NIE and Ss1a produced promising results (Yunus et al., 2019) and was afterwards implemented in a cassette format, but with the inclusion of a single recombinant antigen (NIE) (Noordin et al., 2021). Another group of researchers evaluated two SsIR—ICT, either detecting IgG or IgG4 (Sadaow et al., 2020). Overall, the ICT based on recombinant antigens showed good performance, with 82–91% sensitivity and 84–100% specificity (Sadaow et al., 2020; Noordin et al., 2021; Yunus et al., 2019). Due to these promising preliminary results, and appeal of use, these recombinant antigen-based ICT deserve further evaluation.

5.3 Tests based on antigen detection

5.3.1 Coproantigen tests

The coproantigen tests detect antigen biomarkers present in stool. This method is usually deemed useful to diagnose infections in the pre-patent period (Little et al., 2019), and to differentiate current from previous infections, due to the rapid negativization after treatment. A coproantigen can also be deployed in a point-of-care rapid test format. As for the diagnosis of strongyloidiasis, a few coproantigen ELISAs have been evaluated mostly in experimental studies in rats (Chaves et al., 2015; Nageswaran et al., 1994; Sykes and McCarthy, 2011). A proof of principle study (Sykes and McCarthy, 2011) in humans is also available. The assays were implemented using either anti-*S. venezuelensis* or *S. ratti* IgG. Overall, they proved successful in detecting the target antigens, but further development and studies in humans are needed.

5.3.2 Skin test reaction

Some experimental studies describing diagnosis through skin test reaction have been published. They were based on intradermal injection of extracts retrieved from disrupted larvae from either homologous or heterologous *Strongyloides* species, causing immediate hypersensitivity (Pellegrino et al., 1961; Porto et al., 2001; Neva et al., 2001; Sato et al., 1986). Reduced reactions were observed in individuals with HTLV-1 co-infection (Neva et al., 2001; Porto et al., 2001). No further implementation of such tests has been reported in the last two decades.

6. Molecular diagnosis

The use of nucleic acid amplification tests (NAATs) such as PCR and Loop-Mediated Isothermal Amplification (LAMP) tests for the diagnosis of strongyloidiasis offers several advantages over traditional coprological and serological approaches, in research studies and for clinical diagnostics. Samples may be easily preserved and tested weeks, months, or years after collection. Preserved specimens may be easily transported long distances at ambient temperature, even in adverse tropical environments, and batch tested in the destination laboratory. Preservation of specimens for DNA analysis also eliminates the risk of laboratory acquired infection inherent in working with human faeces, serum and cultured *Strongyloides* larvae (Bradbury and Herwaldt, 2020). However, it must be recognized NAATs are not 100% sensitive or specific for the diagnosis of *S. stercoralis* and there is an absence of clinical validation data for most available NAATs. Furthermore, pre-analytical variables such as method of preservation and method of DNA extraction, and analytical variables, such as the presence of PCR inhibitors in the sample, the quality of PCR reagents, and the efficiency of the PCR cycler employed, can markedly affect the performance of these tests. Although these assays may detect free *S. stercoralis* DNA in faeces in the absence of visible larvae, false negatives also do occur (Verweij et al., 2009).

6.1 PCR assays for *Strongyloides stercoralis*

Several conventional, nested, and real-time PCRs targeting variously portions of the *S. stercoralis 5.8S rRNA*, *18S rRNA*, *28S rRNA*, ITS-1, ITS-2, or DNA repeats in the *S. stercoralis* genome, have been published (Chankongsin et al., 2020; Ghasemikhah et al., 2017; Holt et al., 2017; Kramme et al., 2011; Lodh et al., 2016; Nilforoushan et al., 2007; Pilotte et al., 2016; Repetto et al., 2013; Robertson et al., 2017; Sharifdini et al., 2015; Sitta et al., 2014; Verweij et al., 2009). Few of these are validated against a suitable reference standard. On review, the nested PCR described by Sharafidini et al. (Sharifdini et al., 2015) appears to have the greatest diagnostic sensitivity, but further validation is required. The ease of amplicon contamination leading to false positives when using a nested approach means very comprehensive PCR product contamination precautions must be taken if routine diagnostic use of this assay is intended. Furthermore, in modern diagnostic laboratories, there is a general preference for real-time PCR assays due to their improved sensitivity compared to conventional PCR and capacity to provide at least partial quantification of larval load (Llewellyn et al., 2016). A recent systematic review of the literature revealed that although having high specificity, the sensitivity of PCR many assays was unsatisfactory (Buonfrate et al., 2018b), suggesting that PCR could not be considered superior to other parasitological technique such as Baermann test (Buonfrate et al., 2018b; Chankongsin et al., 2020).

A *Strongyloides* real-time PCR (qPCR) assay developed by Verweij et al. (Verweij et al., 2009), with or without modifications, remains the most comprehensively validated and widely employed NAAT assay in both diagnostic and research laboratories. This assay targets a 101 bp portion of the 18S ribosomal small subunit gene. It should be noted that the target is not specific to *S. stercoralis* and other species of *Strongyloides* will be amplified by this assay, including *S. f. fuelleborni*, *Strongyloides venezuelensis* and *S. ratti* (Saugar et al., 2015; Barratt et al., 2019). Only the Verweij PCR has been used in the testing of dogs. This has been performed in Italy, Australia, Kiribati, and elsewhere (Buonfrate et al., 2017a; Beknazarova et al., 2019, 2020; Zendejas-Heredia et al., 2021) but no diagnostic validation studies have been performed using the assay on faecal samples from this host. It has been demonstrated that the assay will amplify both *cox1* lineages of *S. stercoralis* (lineage A; reported from humans, dogs, cats, and non-human primates, and lineage B; apparently restricted to dogs) (Beknazarova et al., 2019). The assay has not yet been used for the diagnosis of strongyloidiasis in cats or non-human primates. It is not known if it will amplify other canine and feline *Strongyloides* spp., such as *Strongyloides tumefaciens* and *Strongyloides felis*, though it does amplify cryptic *Strongyloides* spp. from Australian dogs (Beknazarova et al., 2019).

Holt et al. (Holt et al., 2017) modified the Verweij PCR by designing an alternative forward primer to improve specificity in their laboratory in the Northern Territory of Australia. This modified version had a 471 bp product. Though the adaptation compared favourably with APC, limited validation was conducted (Holt et al., 2017). Holt's modified forward primer has been employed both in an individual PCR assay, and as part of a five-target multiplex assay targeting three intestinal protozoa, *S. stercoralis* and equine herpes virus (EHV) control (Llewellyn et al., 2016). This assay was determined to be semi-quantitative when tested against dilutions of a plasmid control. When tested against 467 samples from East Timor and 213 from Cambodia, only one PCR positive (from East Timor) was detected. This was despite four of the Cambodian samples having *Strongyloides* larvae detected by microscopy (Llewellyn et al., 2016). Given the known high prevalence of *S. stercoralis* in Cambodia and likely moderate to high prevalence in East Timor, this result is surprising and a comprehensive validation of this PCR is indicated prior to further use. Barda et al. (Barda et al., 2018) also modified the forward primer of the Verweij et al. (Verweij et al., 2009) PCR and conducted validation studies of this modification using Baermann sedimentation on two separate stools as a reference standard. The assay was also clinically validated using two DNA extraction techniques. The method of DNA extraction greatly affected the sensitivity and specificity of the PCR assay (Table 4).

Another *S. stercoralis* qPCR assay was published by Pilotte et al. (Pilotte et al., 2016). This assay adopted a new approach to primer design, by scanning the genome for repetitive elements which could be used as PCR targets. This approach is designed to yield a more sensitive assay due to high copy number repeats being chosen. The assay was validated against a panel of 79 stool samples collected in East Timor and already tested using Holt's primers (Llewellyn et al., 2016), only one of which was positive for *S. stercoralis*. The assay correlated well against this panel, but noting the aforementioned limitations of Holt's assay, a far more robust clinical validation using a high sensitivity reference standard is required. The assay has been used in a small number of parasite prevalence studies (Benjamin-Chung et al., 2021; Bradbury et al., 2020, 2021a).

Table 4 Analytical and pre-analytical variables and calculation of diagnostic performance values[a] for all *Strongyloides* PCR assay validation studies where a high sensitivity coproculture technique was available for use as a reference standard.

PCR assay	n tested (n+ve by reference method)	Source	Preservation method	Preservation time	DNA Extraction method	PCR Target (amplicon size)	Cycling conditions	Inhibition control	Reference Method	Sensitivity (95% CI) (using phenotypic reference standards only)	Specificity (95% CI) (using phenotypic reference standards only)	Sensitivity (95% CI) (using a composite reference standard[a])	Reference
Real-time PCR (Verweij)	212 (54)	Ghana	Frozen or in ethanol[b]	ns	QIAamp Tissue Kit (Qiagen) with pre-heating in 2% polyvinyl-polypyrolidone	*18S rRNA* (101 bp)	95 °C for 15 min, 50 cycles of 95 °C for 15 s, 60 °C for 60 s	Phocince herpesvirus	Baermann & 2 × Modified charcoal coproculture	61.1% (46.9–74.1%)	92.4% (87.1–96.0%)	72.0% (60.4–81.8%)	Verweij et al. (2009)
Real-time PCR (Verweij)	160 (41)	Bangladesh	−20C freezing	1 year	MoBio Powersoil kit	*18S rRNA* (101 bp)	95 °C for 15 min, 50 cycles of 95 °C for 15 s, 60 °C for 30 s, 72 °C for 30 s	Commerical synthetic DNA internal control	3 × Harada-Mori	34.5% (20.1–50.6%)	99.2% (95.4– 100%)	33.3% (19.6–49.6%)	Sultana et al. (2013)
Real-time PCR (Verweij)	501	Cambodia	−20 °C freezing	ns	QIAmp DNA Stool Kit	*18S rRNA* (101 bp)	95 °C for 10 min, 40 cycles of 95 °C for 15 s, 60 °C for 30 s	Spiking duplicate samples with *S. stercoralis 18s rRNA* plasmid control	APC & Baermann	61% (49.6–71.6%)	92.7% (87.8–96.0%)	66.3% (55.9–75.7%)	Schär et al. (2013)
Real-time PCR (Verweij)	466 (85)	Iran	70% ethanol at RT	ns	Phenol–chloroform–isoamyl alcohol extraction with prior rounds of freeze-thawing	*18S rRNA* (101 bp)	95 °C for 10 min, 40 cycles of 95 °C for 15 s, 60 °C for 60 s	None	APC & FEC	84.7% (75.3–91.6%)	95.8% (93.3–97.6%)	75.2% (66.4–82.7%)	Sharifdini et al. (2015)
Real-time PCR (Verweij)	256 (28)	Côte d'Ivoire	70% ethanol	ns	QIAmp DNA Stool Kit	*18S rRNA* (101 bp)	95 °C for 15 min, 40 cycles of 95 °C for 15 s, 60 °C for 30 s	ns	APC & Baermann	50% (30.7–69.3%)	92.5% (88.3–95.6%)	54.39% (40.7–67.6%)	Becker et al. (2015)

Continued

Table 4 Analytical and pre-analytical variables and calculation of diagnostic performance values[a] for all *Strongyloides* PCR assay validation studies where a high sensitivity coproculture technique was available for use as a reference standard.—cont'd

PCR assay	n tested (n+ve by reference method)	Source	Preservation method	Preservation time	DNA Extraction method	PCR Target (amplicon size)	Cycling conditions	Inhibition control	Reference Method	Sensitivity (95% CI) (using phenotypic reference standards only)	Specificity (95% CI) (using phenotypic reference standards only)	Sensitivity (95% CI) (using a composite reference standard[a])	Reference
Real-time PCR (Verweij)	256 (28)	Côte d'Ivoire	70% ethanol	ns	QIAmp DNA Stool Kit	*18S rRNA* (101 bp)	95 °C for 15 min, 50 cycles of 95 °C for 15 s, 60 °C for 60 s	ns	APC & Baermann	70% (45.7–88.1%)	91.2% (86.8–94.6%)	59.7% (45.8–72.4%)	Becker et al. (2015)
Real-time PCR (Verweij)	237 (35)	Argentina, Paraguay, Bolivia, Peru	−20 °C freezing	ns	Overnight in GTES buffer, followed by mechanical disruption and QIAamp DNA Stool Mini Kit extraction	*18S rRNA* (101 bp)	ns	Stools spiked with *Trypanosoma cruzi* culture and *T. cruzi* PCR performed on DNA extract	APC & FEC	100% (90.0–100%)	82.18% (76.2–87.2%)	100% (90.0–100%)	Repetto et al. (2016)
Real-time PCR (Verweij)	223 (20)	Italy (incl. Immigrants & travellers)	Fresh faeces	ns	Roche Magnapure LC.2 with overnight pre-freezing in 2% polyvinyl-polypyrolidone, followed by one round of freze-thaw	*18S rRNA* (101 bp)	95 °C for 15 min, 50 cycles of 95 °C for 15 s, 60 °C for 60 s	Phocince herpesvirus	APC	72.0% (50.6–87.9%)	98.9% (96.4–99.9%)	56.8% (41.0–71.7%)	Buonfrate et al. (2017b)
Real-time PCR (Verweij)	323 (100)	Mozambique	96% ethanol	ns	QIAamp Tissue Kit (Qiagen) with pre-heating in 2% polyvinyl-polypyrolidone followed by proteinase K pre-treatment	*18S rRNA* (101 bp)	95 °C for 15 min, 50 cycles of 95 °C for 15 s, 60 °C for 60 s	Phocince herpesvirus	APC, Baermann, FEC, Direct smear microscopy	88.8% (80.8–94.3%)	77.1% (70.1–82.6%)	92.3% (86.7–96.1%)	Meurs et al. (2017)

Real-time PCR (Verweij)	143 (4)	Colombia	−20°C freezing	ns	ns	*18S rRNA* (101 bp)	ns	TaqMan® Exogenous Internal Positive control (Applied Biosystems)	APC, Harada-Mori, Direct smear microscopy & FEC	75% (20.1–100%)	79.1% (72.0–86.2%)	97.0% (84.2 to 99.9%)	Campo-Polanco et al. (2018)
Real-time PCR (Verweij) - Sybr Green modification	231 (12)	Spain (incl. Immigrants & travellers)	Fresh faeces	ns	QiaAmp DNA stool Mini kit with pre-concentration in Bioparapred-Midi columns	*18S rRNA* (101 bp)	95°C for 15 min, 50 cycles of 95°C for 10 s, 60°C for 30 s, 72°C for 30 s	Spiking duplicate samples with *S. venezuelensis* L3 DNA	3 × Harada-Mori	93.8% (69.8–99.8%)	86.5% (81.2–90.8%)		Saugar et al. (2015)
Real-time PCR (Verweij) - Sybr Green modification	396 (48)	Ethiopia	Fresh faeces at 4°C	ns	QiaAmp DNA stool Mini kit with pre-concentration in Bioparapred-Midi columns	*18S rRNA* (101 bp)	95°C for 15 min, 50 cycles of 95°C for 15 s, 60°C for 10 s, 72°C for 30 s	Spiking duplicate samples with *S. venezuelensis* L3 DNA	Baermann	43.1% (29.4–57.7%)	91% (87.5–57.8%)	97.1% (85.1–99.9%)	Amor et al. (2016)
Real-time PCR (Verweij) in multiplex	193 (46)	Tanzania	−20°C freezing	Between 0 days & 1 year	QIAamp Tissue Kit (Qiagen) with pre-heating in 2% polyvinyl-polypyrolidone	*18S rRNA* (101 bp)	95°C for 15 min, 50 cycles of 95°C for 30 s, 60°C for 30 s, 72°C for 30 s	ns	Baermann	17.39% (7.8–31.4%)	93.9% (88.7–97.2%)	30.9% (19.1–44.8%)	Knopp et al. (2014)
Barda modification of Verweij real-time PCR	95 (69)	Lao PDR	Ethanol[c]	ns	QIAamp Tissue Kit (Qiagen)	*18S rRNA* (184 bp)	50°C for 2 min, 95°C for 10 min, 45 cycles of 95°C for 15 s, 58°C for 60 s	plasmid	2 × Baermann	27.5%	76.9%	31.3% (21.3–42.6%)	Barda et al. (2018)
Barda modification of Verweij real-time PCR	95 (69)	Lao PDR	Ethanol[c]	ns	QIAamp Tissue Kit (Qiagen) with proteinase K pre-treatment	*18S rRNA* (184 bp)	50°C for 2 min, 95°C for 10 min, 45 cycles of 95°C for 15 s, 58°C for 60 s	ns	2 × Baermann	76.8%	65.4%	77.5% (66.8–86.1%)	Barda et al. (2018)

Continued

Table 4 Analytical and pre-analytical variables and calculation of diagnostic performance values[a] for all *Strongyloides* PCR assay validation studies where a high sensitivity coproculture technique was available for use as a reference standard.—cont'd

PCR assay	n tested (n + ve by reference method)	Source	Preservation method	Preservation time	DNA Extraction method	PCR Target (amplicon size)	Cycling conditions	Inhibition control	Reference Method	Sensitivity (95% CI) (using phenotypic reference standards only)	Specificity (95% CI) (using phenotypic reference standards only)	Sensitivity (95% CI) (using a composite reference standard[a])	Reference
Real-time PCR (Chankongsin)	104 (27)	Lao PDR	90% ethanol at RT	ns	QIAamp Tissue Kit (Qiagen) with proteinase K pre-treatment	*28S rRNA* (92 bp)	50 °C for 2 min, 95 °C for 10 min, 45 cycles of 95 °C for 15 s, 58 °C for 60 s	ns	APC, Baermann & Direct smear microscopy	66.8% (46.0–83.5%)	89.6% (80.6–95.4%)	74.3% (56.7–87.5%)	Chankongsin et al. (2020)
Nested PCR (Sharifdini)	466 (85)	Iran	70% ethanol at RT	ns	Phenol–chloroform–isoamyl alcohol extraction with prior rounds of freeze-thawing	*cox1* (Outer: 509 bp, Inner: 261 bp)	Outer: 95 °C for 6 min, 35 cycles of 95 °C for 45 s, 55 °C for 60 s, 72 °C for 60 s, final extension 72 °C for 6 min Inner: 95 °C for 2 min, 25 cycles of 95 °C for 15 s, 60 °C for 30 s, 70 °C for 30 s, final extension 72 °C for 6 min	ns	APC, FEC	100% (95.8–100%)	91.6% (88.4–94.2%)	100% (96.9–100%)	Sharifdini et al. (2015)

Nested PCR (Moghaddassani) using novel outer primers and Nilforoushan (2007) inner primers	46 (16)	Iran	70% ethanol	ns	Modification of QIAamp® DNA stool MiniKit with prior 70% ethanol/ether concentration	ITS 1 to *5.8S rRNA* to ITS 2 region (Outer: 750 bp, Inner: 680 bp)	Outer: 95 °C for 7 min, 30 cycles of 94 °C for 45 s, 55 °C for 90 s, 72 °C for 90 s, final extension 72 °C for 5 min Inner: 94 °C for 3 min, 30 cycles of 94 °C for 45 s, 60 °C for 45 s, 72 °C for 60 s, final extension 72 °C for 5 min	ns	APC	75% (47.6–92.7%)	100% (88.4–100%)	57.1% (34.0–78.2%)	Moghaddassani et al. (2011)
Conventional PCR (Moghaddassani)	46 (16)	Iran	70% ethanol	ns	Modification of QIAamp® DNA stool MiniKit with prior 70% ethanol/ether concentration	ITS 1 to *5.8S rRNA* region (114 bp)	95 °C for 5 min, 30 cycles of 94 °C for 30 s, 58 °C for 45 s, 72 °C for 45 s, final extension 72 °C for 5 min	ns	APC	76.2% (52.8–91.8%)	100% (86.3–100%)	76.2% (52.8–91.8%)	Moghaddassani et al. (2011)

[a] A composite of the results of all methods combined, including the assay being validated. In some cases, this includes additional phenotypic reference methods to those stated in the reference method column.
[b] Diagnostic sensitivities were calculated in this work from data provided in the reference using the reported results of a single or a combination high sensitivity coproculture technique as a reference standard.
[c] Percentage not stated.
GTES Buffer: glycine, Tris/Cl, EDTA, SDS buffer, APC: Agar plate culture; Baermann: Baermann sedimentation; FEC: Formalin-ethyl acetate sedimentation; *18S rRNA*: 18S ribsomal RNA small subunit gene; *cox1*: Cytochrome oxidase 1 gene; ITS 1: Internal Trascribed Spacer 1 gene; ITS 2: Internal Trascribed Spacer 2 gene; ns: not stated.

Chankongsin et al. (Chankongsin et al., 2020) recently described an *S. stercoralis* TaqMan (Thermo Fisher Scientific) qPCR based on the primers originally developed for using a fluorescence energy transfer (FRET) qPCR described by Kramme et al. (Kramme et al., 2011). This was clinically validated in the Lao PDR and found to have a moderate sensitivity (66.8%) when compared to a combination of only APC and Baermann sedimentation as a reference standard.

Commercial multiplex qPCR panels are increasingly being used in diagnostic laboratories. Only one such panel, the The Allplex™ GI-Helminth (I) assay, includes primers for *S. stercoralis*. These primers and their target are commercial-in-confidence. The assay demonstrated an 80.0% sensitivity and 97.3% specificity when tested against a panel of faeces positive for various parasites by microscopy (Autier et al., 2018). This sensitivity was increased to 86% with the addition of a bead-beating step prior to DNA extraction. It should be noted that various techniques had been used individually or in combination to assemble the reference panel. A prospective clinical validation performed in an endemic community and using a high sensitivity reference test would be of benefit to better determine the assay performance characteristics.

Recently, a promising *S. stercoralis* duplex droplet PCR assay has been described. Validation studies of this assay compared to microscopic techniques (FECT and APC) are promising, with a 98% sensitivity and 90% specificity reported. The limit of detection was a single larva and no cross-reactions with other parasites were reported (Iamrod et al., 2021).

6.2 Loop-mediated isothermal amplification (LAMP) assays for *Strongyloides* diagnosis

LAMP assays have advantages over PCR in that they require less complex equipment for performance. By using technology based on polymerases with strand-displacement activity that can amplify nucleic acid under isothermal conditions, equipment is simplified without the need for the cycling reactions of PCR (Watts et al., 2014). There is also the potential to use lyophilized reagents that are stable at room temperature (Watts et al., 2019). Like PCR, stool diagnosis with LAMP also requires highly specific primers due to the presence of DNA from a large number of other sources, including foodstuffs and other organisms (Watts et al., 2014; Verweij et al., 2009). Two LAMP assays have been developed for *Strongyloides* diagnosis (Watts et al., 2014; Fernández-Soto et al., 2016).

The primers developed by Watts et al. (Watts et al., 2014) target a 184 bp region on the 28S ribosomal subunit gene and are comprised of forward and backward outer primers (F3, B3), forward and backward inner primers (FIP, BIP) and a loop primer (LB) to reduce the reaction time. The assay also employed Syto-82 (Life Technologies), to allow visualisation of positive results without opening the reaction tube to reduce the risk of laboratory contamination with amplified product. The analytical specificity of the primer set was tested using human DNA and a range of DNA extracted from gut bacteria, fungi and parasites and 30 *Strongyloides*-negative stool specimens from a low prevalence area (Watts et al., 2014). The analytical sensitivity / limit of detection (LoD) was determined using serial dilutions of a plasmid with target DNA with detection to <10 copies (Watts et al., 2014). Serial dilutions were also made of DNA extracted from negative stool spiked with single *S. ratti* larvae with a LAMP assay limit of detection of 10^{-2} dilution, compared to 10^{-3} for a PCR assay based on the method developed by Verweij et al. (Sultana et al., 2013; Verweij et al., 2009; Watts et al., 2014, 2019).

The Watts et al. (Watts et al., 2014) LAMP assay was also compared to a PCR, based on the method by Verweij et al. (Verweij et al., 2009), in a survey of DNA extracts from three different locations: Dhaka, Sydney and northern Queensland (Watts et al., 2019). Based on the primer design the assay will also detect *Strongyloides* spp. other than *S. stercoralis*, including *S. ratti* (Watts et al., 2014). While concordance with negative results (negative percentage agreement) was 100% with the LAMP and PCR assays, the concordance of positive results (positive percentage agreement) ranged from 91.6% to 71% depending on the source of the DNA extracts (Watts et al., 2019). Using the Verweij et al. (Verweij et al., 2009) PCR as a reference, the total positive percentage agreement was 77.4% (95% CI 63.8–87.7%) and the total negative percentage agreement was 100% (95% CI 98.9–100%). Some of this variation may have been due to DNA degradation in some of the samples and a clinical study that compared freshly extracted stool samples would be valuable. Modifying reagents such as the DNA polymerase may also improve sensitivity. While this assay shows promise, a clinical validation against a high sensitivity phenotypic reference standard such as APC, Baermann sedimentation, or both is still indicated.

The LAMP assay developed by Fernández-Soto et al. (Fernández-Soto et al., 2016) targets a 329 bp region on the 18S ribosomal subunit gene and is comprised of forward and backward outer primers (F3, B3), forward and backward inner primers (FIP, BIP) (Fernández-Soto et al., 2016).

Positive results were confirmed using the addition of SYBR Green (Invitrogen) at the completion of the reaction (Fernández-Soto et al., 2016). On analytical specificity testing, there was no amplification of DNA from a range of gut parasites (Fernández-Soto et al., 2016). The LoD of the LAMP assay was determined using serial dilutions of *S. venezuelensis* larval DNA and was found to be 0.01 ng (Fernández-Soto et al., 2016). This was also the limit of detection for a PCR assay based on the F3 and B3 LAMP primers.

The Fernández-Soto et al. (Fernández-Soto et al., 2016) LAMP assay was effective in detecting *Strongyloides* DNA in urine and stool using a rat model (*S. venezuelensis*). Out of a series of 11 human stool samples, 7 were positive using microscopy-based diagnostics and the LAMP assay (Fernández-Soto et al., 2016). Subsequently, urine from 24 individuals diagnosed with strongyloidiasis on the basis of microscopy-based methods or serology were tested with the LAMP assay and the PCR assay based on the F3 and B3 primers (Fernández-Soto et al., 2020). Twelve of the 24 urine samples were positive using the LAMP assay and all were negative on the PCR assay (Fernández-Soto et al., 2020). A cause of the discrepancy may be that the PCR reaction was inhibited by protein in the urine and the LAMP assay was less affected (Fernández-Soto et al., 2020). Further development of the LAMP assay would include additional analytical specificity testing using DNA extracted from gut bacteria and fungi (Fernández-Soto et al., 2016) and clinical validation studies.

6.3 NAAT testing on non-stool specimens (urine, respiratory samples, serum, cerebral spinal fluid)

A number of preliminary studies have investigated the diagnosis of strongyloidiasis using urine, respiratory specimens and serum. In terms of urine specimens, Fernández-Soto et al. (Fernández-Soto et al., 2020) used a LAMP assay to detect *S. stercoralis* DNA in urine from 12 of 24 patients diagnosed with strongyloidiasis either by FECT, APC or serology (also see the *Loop-mediated isothermal amplification (LAMP) assays for Strongyloides Diagnosis* section of this review). Serology positive patients had the poorest correlation (Fernández-Soto et al., 2020). This study also used a touchdown PCR based on the LAMP primers and applied this to positive patient's urine samples, while the assay amplified *S. venezuelensis* DNA, it did not yield a product in any urine samples tested (Fernández-Soto et al., 2020).

Use of the Verweij et al. (Verweij et al., 2009) qPCR on urine and faeces had better correlation, with urine yielding slightly less positives than faeces (Formenti et al., 2019). Lodh et al. (Lodh et al., 2016) developed a conventional PCR targeting a DNA-repeats and with a 125 bp product. This was applied to testing faeces and urine of people from an endemic area of Argentina. The analysis of urine yielded almost double the number of positive results when compared to faecal analysis. As the authors acknowledge, more validation is required before the meaning of these results can be accurately interpreted.

To demonstrate proof-of-concept, microscopy-positive broncho-alveolar lavage (BAL) fluid was positive for *Strongyloides* on a PCR based on the Verweij et al. (Verweij et al., 2009) method and the Watts et al. (Watts et al., 2014) LAMP assay, after DNA was extracted using the High Pure DNA template preparation kit (Roche) (Watts et al., 2019). Some serum samples from broncho-alveolar lavage and stool microscopy-positive persons were also positive using these assays, following serum DNA extraction using the NucliSENS easyMag system (bioMerieux), however, further validation for these specimen types, including analytical and clinical sensitivity testing is required.

Gorgani-Firouzjaee et al. (Gorgani-Firouzjaee et al., 2018) also used their conventional adaptation of the Verweij et al. (Verweij et al., 2009) qPCR to screen the serum of immunosuppressed patients and compare this to microscopy and APC of their faecal samples. A sixfold higher number of positives were detected in the serum samples, but only five were sequenced (it is not stated if these five were from any of the six positives by coprological methods) and a *cox1* conventional genotyping target PCR yielded no amplification in the same DNA extracts (Gorgani-Firouzjaee et al., 2018).

The Verweij PCR has been employed to detect and diagnose *S. stercoralis* infection in individual patient sputum (Beknazarova et al., 2019). The Saugar SYBR Green modification of the Verweij PCR was used to simultaneously detected *S. stercoralis* DNA in BAL fluid, cerebrospinal fluid (CSF), serum, and tissue biopsies from the duodenum, stomach, oesophagus and bone marrow of an HIV positive patient with disseminated strongyloidiasis and multi-organ failure, leading to appropriate treatment and recovery (Le Pogam et al., 2020).

It is important not to interpret positive results by NAAT in the absence of a positive reference test result as indicative of higher sensitivity of NAAT assay when used in urine, fluid, sputum, or serum matrices unless comprehensive validations are conducted to support this assumption. Validation studies should include an analytical specificity testing including faecal, urethral and vaginal flora which may be found contaminating urine in small quantities. The difficulties in interpreting comparison studies of PCR assays on urine, serum and faeces highlight the need for proper validation of assays prior to use in research or diagnostics.

6.4 Pre-analytical variables in NAAT testing

As important as choice of NAAT assay for diagnostic use is the choice of preservation and DNA extraction method. NAATs may be performed on any sample preserved in a way that maintains DNA integrity. It should be noted that formalin cross-links, fragments and base modifies DNA and is thus not an appropriate preservative for use in NAAT testing. DNA extraction from stool requires an efficient nucleic acid extraction process due to reaction inhibitors, for example, humic and tannic acids and nucleases, and the intermittent larval output in chronic infection (Dreyer et al., 1996; Watts et al., 2019). The same pre-analytical variables which affect PCR also affect LAMP testing.

Faeces and other tissue and fluids for *S. stercoralis* PCR testing have previously been extracted from fresh faeces or faeces variously preserved by storage by freezing at −20 °C (Campo-Polanco et al., 2018), −80 °C (Bradbury et al., 2021a), 100% ethanol (Robertson et al., 2017), 96% ethanol (Meurs et al., 2017), 70% ethanol (Becker et al., 2015), Zymo DNA/RNA Shield (Zymo Research) (Zendejas-Heredia et al., 2021), 5% KCr_2 (Llewellyn et al., 2016) and dimethyl sulfoxide, disodium EDTA with saturated NaCl (DESS) (Beknazarova et al., 2017). Beknazarova et al. (Beknazarova et al., 2017) compared DESS at a ratio of 1:1 and 1:3 with neat dog faeces spiked with larvae of *S. ratti* and stored at room temperature. DNA was extracted using the PowerSoil kit (Qiagen) then subjected to the Verweij qPCR. PCR products were detected for all samples with a slightly lower Ct for unpreserved faeces at day 0 (average Ct 16 vs Ct 18 for DESS preserved samples, possibly a due to the dilution effect of the preservative), after 56 days, but those stored in DESS had an on average 5 points lower Ct in the PCR. No other validation studies have been performed on the efficacy of these various preservation methods and it cannot be assumed that preservation validation studies for other soil-transmitted helminths (STH) (Ayana et al., 2019), which are passed as eggs, will have corresponding efficacy for the preservation of *Strongyloides* larvae. Similarly, no other studies have been performed regarding the effect of time in storage on NAAT assay results for *Strongyloides*.

Commercial fixatives such as Total-Fix (Medical Chemical Corporation) and EcoFix (Cardinal Health) are now commonly used in U.S. laboratories performing multiplex PCR assays, but these also have not been validated in comparison trials.

The choice of DNA extraction method will also impact the results of NAAT testing. A major consideration when performing NAATs on faeces is the presence of PCR inhibitors in the sample matrix. Kits designed for soil or faecal extraction generally are superior for removal of such inhibitors than tissue or blood extraction kits, though the latter may be more effective when dealing with samples of sputum, fluid, or tissue for *Strongyloides* NAAT testing. One comparison study has been performed on DNA extraction kits for *Strongyloides* testing using the Verweij PCR (Sultana et al., 2013). This study employed human faeces spiked with between 1 and 10 larvae of *S. ratti*. It compared Qiagen PowerSoil kit (now superseded by the Qiagen PowerFecal Pro kit), the Ultra Clean Faecal DNA kit (MoBio Laboratories,) with prior bead beating, a modification of the QiaAmp Tissue kit (Qiagen,) incorporating polyvinylpolypyrrolidone pre-treatment, and the NucliSens EasyMag (bioMerieux) automated DNA extraction platform withprior bead beating. This study found that the MoBio PowerSoil kit led to the greatest analytical sensitivity based on a model of *S. ratti* spiked into stool (Sultana et al., 2013). Barda et al. (Barda et al., 2018) compared DNA extraction in the QiaAmp kit with and without pre-treatment in proteinase K using their modification of the Verweij qPCR and found much improved sensitivity using proteinase K pre-treatment (Barda et al., 2018). Fernández-Soto et al. (Fernández-Soto et al., 2016) used a Bioparapred-Midi column (Leti Diagnostics) to concentrate the stool pellet prior to DNA extraction. Several other DNA extraction protocols have been employed in various studies (Table 4), but without comparison to other methods.

6.5 Analytical variables

The assay described by Verweij et al. (Verweij et al., 2009), sometimes with minor variations, remains the most thoroughly validated assay, with 10 clinical validation studies employing sensitive reference standards having been published (Table 4). Many of these papers report a wide range of sensitivity and specificity results, which may be attributable to variations pre-analytical and analytical processes more than variables in the populations studied. When used as a qPCR with the primers and probe designed by Verweij et al.

(Verweij et al., 2009) and validated against an optimal reference standard (Baermann sedimentation or APC), this assay was has demonstrated sensitivities ranging between 34.5% and 100% and a specificities of between 77.1% and 98.9% when compared to phenotypic tests (Table 4). The wide variation in assay performance may be attributed to not just the sampled cohort and pre-analytical variables, but also to a surprising array of modifications to the cycling conditions and Ct value cut-offs employed. One such modification has been the use of the Verweij et al. primers (Verweij et al., 2009) but with SYBR green (Invitrogen) instead of Taqman probes for amplicon detection (Saugar et al., 2015). The Verweij et al. (Verweij et al., 2009) primers have also been used in a conventional PCR form, though without validation (Gorgani-Firouzjaee et al., 2018). Although the primers employed are the same, such changes in analytical processes may impact sensitivity and specificity. Reagent storage and quality and the PCR cycler used, and the frequency of maintenance, may also influence on assay performance. These observations apply to other examples where NAAT tests have been used by different groups.

Given the variability in sample preservation, DNA extraction, primers, PCR cycling conditions and reference standards employed, it is difficult to determine the true sensitivity and specificity of many NAAT tests for *S. stercoralis*. Even the most widely validated assay, the Verweij et al. (Verweij et al., 2009) real time PCR, can yield vastly different values depending on these variables. This makes comparison of data from different trials and population surveys difficult. Standardisation of NAAT testing protocols for *S. stercoralis* would greatly benefit the WHO 2030 goals for the for the implementation of control strategies for this parasite (Montresor et al., 2020) by allowing comparability of survey data. A thorough validation of all assays, including pre-analytical variables, is necessary to determine what the optimal molecular testing approach for the detection of *S. stercoralis* infection is. This will be necessary if the results of such assays are used to guide interventions.

6.6 Quantification of larval Output by PCR

Unlike PCR for bacterial or viral infections, where millions or billions of copies of the pathogen genome may be extracted in a single specimen, there is often a very low number of individual parasitic elements in faeces (Dreyer et al., 1996). When performing Baermann sedimentation or APC, large amounts (often >1 g) of stool are used. However, most commercial DNA extraction kits recommend using only 250 mg of stool. As larval numbers in faeces are often low and larvae are not equally distributed throughout the specimen, this presents a risk of sampling error.

Some authors have suggested qPCR as a semi-quantitative approach to determining larval load (Llewellyn et al., 2016). A low Ct on qPCR may suggest high numbers of excreted larvae and possibly indicate hyper-infection. However, outside of this scenario and unlike egg excretion for other STH, larval excretion in strongyloidiasis is intermittent (Dreyer et al., 1996; Page et al., 2018) and therefore unreliable as a measure of parasite load. Moreover, the autoinfective cycle of *S. stercoralis* means that the intensity of infection can vary with the host's immune status (Page et al., 2018). Another important consideration is that the more developed L3 and free-living adult stages will yield higher quantities of DNA. The effect of worm development on quantification results in PCRs for other STH has been discussed in depth elsewhere (Papaiakovou et al., 2019). Stool which has not been preserved promptly after passage is not ideal for such quantification approaches (Papaiakovou et al., 2019).

6.7 Quality control and quality assurance

Quality control is imperative to any NAAT testing. For example, reagents need to be in-date, staff need to be appropriately trained, and equipment maintained and monitored. Non-template and inhibition controls must be performed, particularly given the large number of inhibitors present in stool. Samples not yielding an amplicon for the inhibition control should be excluded from analysis in research studies, or another sample collected and testing repeated in the context of diagnostic use.

Where therapy will be administered as part of a research study, treatment program or routine clinical care, it is essential from an ethical standpoint that the diagnostic tests used are appropriately validated and that there an ongoing process of test quality assurance and laboratory accreditation. The Dutch Foundation for Quality Assessment in Medical Laboratories (SKML) offers a The Helminth External Molecular Quality Assessment Scheme (HEMQAS) (SKML) which includes *S. stercoralis*. The Royal College of Pathologists of Australasia Quality Assurance Program (RCPA QAP) is also currently investigating the feasibility of a QAP for *Strongyloides* nucleic acid tests (Watts, personal communication, 2022).

Where laboratories cannot access an external quality assurance scheme (EQAS), periodic blinded testing within a laboratory and blinded interlaboratory specimen exchange are alternative approaches to quality assurance.

6.8 Validation

The most pressing issue for the diagnosis of, and population screening for, strongyloidiasis is the need for appropriate analytical and clinical validation of tests prior to their use. This is particularly important if test results will form the basis for treatment. Examples of guidelines for the laboratory (analytical) validation of tests are published by the FDA and the CLSI (FDA., Garrett et al., 2008) (US Food and Drug Administration, 2017; CLSI, 2008). The STARD Guidelines provide a framework for the clinical evaluation of diagnostic tests (Cohen et al., 2016).

Any validation approach should include the complete sample preservation, transport, and DNA extraction approach. Many publications of prevalence studies have employed either unvalidated assays or the Verweij PCR but using alternative pre-analytical processes which may alter the reported sensitivity and specificity of that test (Table 4). Cases of amplification in samples not found to contain *S. stercoralis* by other methods should not be attributed to improved sensitivity of the PCR used without reference to the comprehensive analytical specificity testing of the assay. Analytical validation in silico using sequences from DNA sequence databases is insufficient. Examples of *Strongyloides* PCR assays amplifying non-target eukaryotic elements in faeces, including *Blastocystis* spp., other helminths, yeasts, and even human genes exist (Sitta et al., 2014; Robertson et al., 2017). Many reported assays have had some form of in vitro analytical validation performed, but the number and breadth of organisms tested for analytical specificity and the choice of template for analytical specificity vary greatly (Table 5).

The absence of a single high sensitivity and reference standard for the detection of *S. stercoralis* infection complicates validation studies. A frustrating approach used in many validation reports is the application of a composite reference standard which includes the test being validated for statistical analysis of sensitivity and specificity. This approach will always yield 100% specificity for the test being validated as there can be no false positives. The approach is based on the assumption that all positives from a NAAT assay are true positives—an assumption for which there is not valid scientific basis. The most accurate measurements of clinical sensitivity and specificity

Table 5 Analytical validation data for all *Strongyloides* PCR and LAMP assay validation studies.

Assay	Analytical sensitivity (limit of detection)	Analytical specificity testing	References
Verweij real-time PCR	10^{-2} *S. stercoralis* DNA extract (life stage and number used not stated)	PARASITES: *Ancylostoma caninum, Ancylostoma duodenale, Angiostrongylus cantonensis, Ascaris lumbricoides, Cryptosporidium hominis, Cryptosporidium parvum Cyclospora cayetanensis, Dientamoeba fragilis, Enterocytozoon bieneusi, Encephalitozoon intestinalis, Entamoeba dispar, Entamoeba histolytica, Faciola hepatica, Giardia duodenalis, Necator americanus, Oesophagostomum bifurcum, Schistosoma mansoni, Taenia saginata, Trichostrongylus vitrinus, Trichuris trichiura* BACTERIA: *Bacillus cereus, Bacteroides fragilis, Campylobacter jejuni, Campylobacter upsaliensis, Clostridioides difficile, Klebsiella aerogenes, Enterococcus faecalis, Escherichia coli* O:157, *Mycobacterium tuberculosis, Proteus mirabilis, Pseudomonas aeruginosa, Salmonella* Enteritidis, *Salmonella* Typhimurium, *Shigella boydii, Shigella dysenteriae, Shigella flexneri, Shigella sonnei, Staphylococcus aureus, Yersinia enterocolitica,* FUNGI: *Aspergillus flavus, Aspergillus fumigatus, Candida albicans, Candida glabrata, Candida krusei, Candida parapsilosis, Candida tropicalis,*	Verweij et al. (2009) and Sultana et al. (2013)
Verweij real-time PCR	ns	PARASITES: *A. duodenale, N. americanus, Ascaris suum, Dirofilaria immitis, Echinococcus granulosus, Loa loa, S. Mansoni, Toxocara canis, Trichinella spiralis, T. trichiura, Wuchereria bancrofti* BACTERIA: Nil FUNGI: Nil	Schär et al. (2016)

Continued

Table 5 Analytical validation data for all *Strongyloides* PCR and LAMP assay validation studies.—cont'd

Assay	Analytical sensitivity (limit of detection)	Analytical specificity testing	References
Verweij real-time PCR	0.1 pg of DNA of *S. venezuelensis* L3 larva DNA	PARASITES: *Anisakis simplex, C. parvum, E. dispar, E. histolytica, G. duodenalis,* hookworm (species not stated), *L. loa, T. saginata, T. spiralis, T. trichura, S. mansoni, W. bancrofti* BACTERIA: Nil FUNGI: Nil	Saugar et al. (2015)
Verweij real-time PCR	10^{-4} dilution of DNA of one *S. stercoralis* L3 larva	PARASITES: *A. lumbricoides, Blastocystis* sp., *Cryptosporidium* sp., *Cystoisospora belli, Dicrocoelium dendriticum, Entamoeba coli, E. histolytica, Enterobius vermicularis, E. bieneusi, Fasciola hepatica, G. duodenalis, Hymenolepis nana, Rhabditis axei, T. saginata, Trichostrongylus* sp., BACTERIA: Nil FUNGI: *Candida albicans*	Sharifdini et al. (2015)
Modification of Verweij real-time PCR	ns	PARASITES: *A. lumbricoides, Blastocystis* sp., *Cryptosporidium* spp., *Cyclospora* sp., *E. coli, E. dispar, Entamoeba hartmanni, E. histolytica, Entamoeba moshkovskii, Endolimax nana, G. duodenalis, Iodamoeba bütschlii, S. mansoni* BACTERIA: Nil FUNGI: Nil	Barda et al. (2018)
Pilotte real-time PCR	10 fg/μL of *S. stercoralis* genomic DNA (initial volume input and life stage not stated)	PARASITES: *A. Lumbricoides, Ancylostoma duodenale, N. americanus, T. trichiura* BACTERIA: *E. coli* FUNGI: Nil	Pilotte et al. (2016)

Chankongsin Real-time PCR	S. stercoralis DNA plasmid control and extracted DNA from S. stercoralis. Results not reported.	PARASITES: *Blastocystis* sp., *Chilomastix mesnili, Cryptosporidium* sp., *C. cayetanensis, C. belli, D. fragilis, Encephalitozoon hellen, E. coli, E. dispar, E. hartmanni, E. histolytica, E. moshkovskii, G. duodenalis, H. nana, I. bütschlii, S. mansoni, Taenia* spp., *Trichostrongylus* spp. BACTERIA: Nil FUNGI: Nil	
Verweij primers as a conventional PCR[a]	One *S. stercoralis* L3 larva $\times 10^{-2}$/g stool when DNA extracted by in house method[a] One *S. stercoralis* L3 larva $\times 10^{-1}$/g stool when DNA extracted by QIAamp DNA Stool Mini Kit	PARASITES: *A. lumbricoides, Blastocystis* sp., *Cryptosporidium* sp., *C. belli, Taenia* sp., *G. duodenalis*, hookworm (species not stated), *H. nana, T. trichiura* BACTERIA: *Salmonella enterica, S. aureus, P. aeruginosa* FUNGI: *C. albicans* VIRUSES: Rotavirus	Repetto et al. (2013)
Repetto conventional PCR[a]	One *S. stercoralis* L3 larva $\times 10^{-2}$/g stool when DNA extracted by in house method[a] One *S. stercoralis* L3 larva/g stool when DNA extracted by QIAamp DNA Stool Mini Kit	PARASITES: *A. lumbricoides, Blastocystis* sp., *C. belli, Cryptosporidium* sp., *G. duodenalis*, hookworm (species not stated), *H. nana, Taenia* sp., *T. trichiura* BACTERIA: *S. enterica, S. aureus, P. aeruginosa* FUNI: *C. albicans* VIRUSES: Rotavirus	Repetto et al. (2013)

Continued

Table 5 Analytical validation data for all *Strongyloides* PCR and LAMP assay validation studies.—cont'd

Assay	Analytical sensitivity (limit of detection)	Analytical specificity testing	References
Sharifdini Nested PCR	10^{-3} dilution of DNA of one *S. stercoralis* filariform larva	PARASITES: *A. lumbricoides, Blastocystis* sp., *Cryptosporidium* sp., *C. Belli, D. dendriticum, E. coli, E. histolytica, E. vermicularis, E. bieneusi, F. hepatica, G. duodenalis, H. nana, R. axei, T. saginata, Trichostrongylus* sp. BACTERIA: Nil FUNGI: *C. albicans*	Sharifdini et al. (2015)
Moghaddassani conventional PCR	ns	PARASITES: *E. coli, E. histolytica, G. duodenalis, H. Nana, Trichostrongylus colubriformis* BACTERIA: *E. coli, Citrobacter* sp. FUNGI: *C. albicans*	Moghaddassani et al. (2011)
Moghaddassani Nested PCR	ns	PARASITES: *H. nana, E. coli, E. histolytica, G. duodenalis, T. colubriformis,* BACTERIA: *E. coli, Citrobacter* sp. FUNGI: *C. albicans* VIRUSES: Nil	Moghaddassani et al. (2011)
Holt modification of Verweij real-time PCR	ns	PARASITES: Nil BACTERIA: Nil FUNGI: Nil VIRUSES: Nil	Holt et al. (2017)
Holt modification of Verweij real-time PCR in multiplex	At least 10^{-7} dilution of a plasmid DNA control (concentration not specified)	PARASITES: *Ascaris* spp., *Cryptosporidium* spp., *E. dispar, E. histolytica, G. duodenalis*, hookworm (species not stated), *T. trichiura,* BACTERIA: Nil FUNGI: Nil	Llewellyn et al. (2016)

Ghasemikhah conventional PCR	ns	PARASITES: *G. duodenalis, H. nana, T. colubriformis.* BACTERIA: Nil FUNGI: Nil	
Watts LAMP		PARASITES: *A. caninum, A. cantonensis, A. lumbricoides, Blastocystis* sp., *C. parvum, D. fragilis, E. vermicularis, F. hepatica, G. duodenalis, N. americanus, S. japonicum, T. saginata, T. trichiura.* BACTERIA: *B. cereus, B. fragilis, C. jejuni, Citrobacter freundii, C. difficile, E. faecalis, E. coli, M. tuberculosis, P. mirabilis, S.* Typhimurium, *S. sonnei, S. aureus, Vibrio cholerae, Vibrio parahaemolyticus, Y. enterocolitica.* FUNGI: *A. flavus, A. fumigatus, C. albicans, C. glabrata, C. krusei, C. parapsilosis, C. tropicalis, Cryptococcus neoformans, Penicillium chrysogenum.*	Watts et al. (2014)
Fernández-Soto LAMP		PARASITES: *A. simplex, Brugia pahangi, C. parvum, Calicophoron daubneyi, D. dendriticum, Echinostoma caproni, E. granulosus, E. histolytica, F. hepatica, G. duodenalis,* hookworm (species not stated), *Hymenolepis diminuta, L. loa, Plasmodium malariae, Plasmodium ovale, Plasmodium vivax, Schistosoma bovis, Schistosoma haematobium, Schistosoma intercalatum, Schistosoma japonicum, Schistosoma mansoni, T. saginata, Taenia taeniformis, T. spiralis,* BACTERIA: Nil FUNGI: Nil	Fernández-Soto et al. (2016)

[a]DNA isolated by incubation in glycine, Tris/Cl, EDTA, SDS (GTES) buffer, followed by three rounds of freeze-thawing, then incubation in nematode lysis buffer, followed by phenol/chloroform/isoamyl alcohol extraction.

would be in those studies that used more than one sensitive coprological larval recovery method for the detection of *Strongyloides* in stool. Specifically, we recommend a combination of Baermann sedimentation and APC, in the hands of experienced parasite morphologists who can easily differentiate *Strongyloides* larvae from those of other helminths.

At a minimum, eight important validation procedures that should be adhered to by all developing new diagnostic PCR assays. These validation conditions are:

a) The novel PCR products should be sequenced to confirm that that the true target is being amplified.

b) The optimal cycling conditions should be determined by testing in a temperature gradient against a positive clinical sample of known DNA concentration.

c) The limit of detection (analytical sensitivity) of the assay should be determined using the nucleic acid extraction method that will be used in testing

d) The novel PCR should always be validated for analytical specificity against a panel of organisms likely to be present in the tested sample matrix (e.g. urine, faeces, soil, food).

e) The novel PCR should be validated against a panel of clinical samples containing the target pathogen.

f) A panel of known negative clinical samples of the same sample type should be analysed to confirm specificity and the absence of false positives.

g) A prospective, blinded, clinical validation study of the assay should be performed in an endemic population, using a highly reliable reference assay or composite reference standard as a comparator.

h) Unusual or unexpected positive amplification by the novel PCR during these validations should always be regarded as a potential 'false positive' unless the positive result is supported by sequence analysis

Only when the above requirements have been met can a diagnostic NAAT assay for *S. stercoralis* (or any other target organism) be considered valid. Thus far, the only assay which meets most of these requirements is the Verweij et al. (Verweij et al., 2009) qPCR, or versions with minor modifications. Although other published PCRs may have similar, or even superior, performance characteristics, these have not been fully validated and thus all results generated using these assays should be interpreted with caution.

6.9 Statistical analysis of validation data

The calculation of disease prevalence in a population may be greatly affected by the choice of test used. To correct for these deficiencies, Bayesian statistical modelling has been applied to estimate disease prevalence (Black and Craig, 2002; Dendukuri and Joseph, 2001; Dendukuri et al., 2010; Stamey et al., 2005; Joseph et al., 1995). These approaches take into consideration the limitations of morphological (reference standard) identification of larvae for *Strongyloides* diagnosis, that increasing the range of tests in a study (e.g. microscopic methods and PCR) will give a closer approximation to the true prevalence and that test results are not independent (Dendukuri et al., 2010). Software has been developed to facilitate the calculation of study sample size based on the number of tests and such technology could be applied to epidemiological research (Dendukuri et al., 2010).

7. Diagnosing *S. stercoralis* infection in domestic animals

S. stercoralis affects not only humans and non-human primates but also dogs, wild canids and cats (Monteiro et al., 2016; Nyambura Njuguna et al., 2017; Wulcan et al., 2019; Ko et al., 2020).

Among *Strongyloides* species infecting companion animals and large livestock, *S. stercoralis* is the only species considered potentially zoonotic (Thamsborg et al., 2017). The only other species having a zoonotic potential is *S. f. fuelleborni,* which infects wild non-human primates. Attempts to find an animal reservoir for *S. f. kellyi* in New Guinea have thus far been unfruitful (Bradbury, 2021).

In dogs, *S. stercoralis* occurs worldwide with prevalence from 0% to 50%, with most studies indicating <5% (Thamsborg et al., 2017). Infection in dogs, as in humans, is considered common/endemic in tropical and subtropical regions, although epidemiological data from low income countries are limited (Gonçalves et al., 2007; Schär et al., 2014; Jaleta et al., 2017). In Europe, prevalence data and data from case reports and case series have been recently reviewed by Ottino and colleagues (Ottino et al., 2020). Sporadic canine infections have been described in numerous countries, with identified hot spots in southern Italy (Paradies et al., 2017), Slovakia (Štrkolcová et al., 2017) and Australia (Beknazarova et al., 2017).

In dogs, *S. stercoralis* infection represents both a veterinary clinical issue and a public health challenge, because in some dogs the infection can induce severe symptoms and can be fatal, and the potential role of dogs (and cats?) in the transmission to humans is a matter of concern. Thus, the role of diagnosis is crucial both in clinical practice and in epidemiological surveys.

7.1 Diagnosis of strongyloidiasis in dogs, in clinical practice

In dogs *S. stercoralis* infection can cause mild to severe symptoms, mostly affecting the gastrointestinal tract (Dillard et al., 2007; Paradies et al., 2017) but pulmonary and dermatological signs have also been described (Cervone et al., 2016; Dashchenko et al., 2020). Associated changes in haematological and biochemical indices (anaemia, leucocytosis, eosinophilia, increased acute phase proteins) could help including the infection in the list of differential diagnosis in dogs with compatible signs, but they are not specific and not constant. The absence of eosinophilia does not exclude strongyloidiasis (Paradies et al., 2017).

A correct diagnosis in clinical practice is crucial also considering that the infection does not respond to commonly used deworming drugs for dogs (such as tetrahydropyridines); oral ivermectin is recommended (Paradies et al., 2019; Yang et al., 2013). No evidence is available in the literature about the widely sponsored use of a deworming spot-on formulation containing moxidectin for prevention and treatment of parasitic infections to treat strongyloidiasis. It is possible that the use of such formulation may hamper the diagnosis without being effective in controlling the infection due to a possible reduction in the parasite load.

The Baermann test remains the most used method for the diagnosis of *S. stercoralis* infection in veterinary practice. In most case reports and case series published in literature (Basso et al., 2019; Cervone et al., 2016; Cvetkovikj et al., 2018; Dillard et al., 2007; Paradies et al., 2017; Eydal and Skirnisson, 2016; Schnyder et al., 2022) definitive diagnosis was reached using Baermann sedimentation. A direct faecal smear may be useful to diagnose the infection in severely affected dogs (Paradies et al., 2017; Cvetkovikj et al., 2018).

The possibility of false negative results using Baermann test in clinical practice has been documented, and the need of other tests to support the diagnosis already suggested (Paradies et al., 2017). The larval output is irregular and may be low (Siddiqui and Berk, 2001). Even dogs with severe clinical signs may yield a negative result in a single test (Paradies et al., 2017). Furthermore, Baermann sedimentation is not routinely employed in clinical practice and larvae could be incorrectly identified as *Angiostrongylus vasorum* (Hall et al., 2020). Thus, the possibility that even cases of patent strongyloidiasis remain undiagnosed in clinical practice is not negligible due to the lack of rapid and efficacious diagnostic methods.

Beside their specific limitations, serological tests and PCR (see below) are not commercially available for veterinary use, thus they are not routinely used in clinics. Unfortunately, rapid diagnostic tests, as recently evaluated in the context of human infection (Balachandra et al., 2021) are not available and/or validated in dogs. These snap tests could be very useful in clinical practice and their development and validation for use in dogs need to be developed because the current assays rely on anti-human IgG antibodies for positive result development.

Post-mortem diagnosis in affected animals could be reached by means of intestinal scarification and microscopic identification of all *S. stercoralis* stages. The histopathology on intestinal biopsies documents the presence of an inflammatory disease (i.e. lymphoplasmacellular enteritis) and could reveal the presence of larvae, ova and adult females mostly in the duodenum gland crypt. Practitioners must be aware that histology from in vivo endoscopic biopsy in dogs with gastrointestinal signs could not reveal the infection in some cases (Paradies, not published data), thus a negative biopsy does not exclude the diagnosis and other tests need to be used in the diagnostic plan in these dogs. The possibility that biopsy could not reveal the infection in some cases was reported also in humans (Mittal et al., 2009; Montes et al., 2010).

In cats *S. stercoralis* infection was recently associated to colonic epithelial grossly, multifocal nodules evidenced at post-mortem examination in which the parasites were localized (Wulcan et al., 2019). Morphologically similar nodules were previously associated to *S. tumefaciences* but it is possible to hypothesise that a misdiagnosis of species could have occurred in the past based on morphology alone.

7.2 Diagnostic tests used for epidemiological surveys

Epidemiological surveys aimed at estimating the prevalence of parasitic infections (including strongyloidiasis) in dogs have been carried out with different coprological methods, including the Baermann concentration method (Iatta et al., 2019; Paradies et al., 2017; Sauda et al., 2018), flotation

(Mircean et al., 2012; Riggio et al., 2013; Zanzani et al., 2014), FLOTAC (Wright et al., 2016), FECT (Eydal and Skirnisson, 2016) (Papazahariadou et al., 2007) and APC (Štrkolcová et al., 2017). Regardless, it is known that *S. stercoralis* is frequently undetected in parasitological surveys for various reasons, such as the intermittent larval shedding and low parasite burden. Moreover, the deployment of tests with low sensitivity for this parasite (such as flotation) further contributes to an underestimation of its prevalence.

7.3 Differences between diagnosis in humans and in dogs

One of the most important differences in the diagnostic approach to *S. stercoralis* infection in humans and dogs is that in humans the risk of missed diagnosis is not acceptable, because the infection is long-lasting due to autoinfection and potentially fatal at any time during life (due to hyperinfection). Thus, in humans, the use of the most sensitive diagnostic techniques to exclude the infection is mandatory. Serology, which has shown the highest sensitivity, has been suggested for screening at population and individual level in this context (Albonico et al., 2016; Buonfrate et al., 2018a; Requena-Méndez et al., 2017), while PCR could be a valid option as a confirmatory test in case of positive serology or for the screening of immunosuppressed patients for whom the sensitivity of serology decreases (Buonfrate et al., 2018b). Conversely, in dogs the infection can be self- limiting, and autoinfection/hyperinfection is not common (Thamsborg et al., 2017), thus the use of a highly-sensitivity but low specificity test for screening could be questionable.

As in humans, serology has higher sensitivity. In studies where more than one diagnostic method has been used for the diagnosis of *S. stercoralis* infection, the prevalence of the infection recorded by serology using IFAT or ELISA was higher than that estimated by Baermann (Júnior et al., 2006; Gonçalves et al., 2007). In the prevalence study by Strkolcova et al. (Štrkolcová et al., 2017) the seroprevalence was 55% compared to a prevalence of 10% at faecal detection. An in-house IFAT, routinely used for *S. stercoralis* diagnosis in humans and showing good performance in dogs (Buonfrate et al., 2017a) resulted the most sensitive test in a study comparing the accuracy of serological, molecular and coprological tests (Iatta et al., 2019). This IFAT resulted more sensitive than the commercial ELISA based on somatic antigens from *S. ratti* larvae for the diagnosis of canine strongyloidiasis (Buonfrate et al., 2017a; Iatta et al., 2019; Paradies et al., 2017). The specificity of IFAT increases with titres >1:320 in dogs (Iatta et al., 2019).

It is not known if *Strongyloides* serology in dogs seroreverts to negative within 18 months following treatment, as it has been observed in human infections (Kearns et al., 2017). Therefore, the clinical significance of positive serology in dogs remains unknown. This aspect must be considered in dogs where the infection is frequently self-limiting. Furthermore, no data are available on the persistence of antibodies after natural elimination of the infection but it has been demonstrated that serology can remain positive for 13 months after treatment (Paradies et al., 2019). Other intrinsic limitations for performing IFAT in dogs are the difficulty in setting up the test and the lack of validation in dogs.

Molecular methods had never been applied in dogs until 2017. The Verweij qPCR (Verweij et al., 2009) was first evaluated in dogs by Buonfrate et al. (Buonfrate et al., 2017a) and demonstrated good performance. A recent survey of dogs in remote Aboriginal communities in northern Australia using the same qPCR found a high prevalence (Beknazarova et al., 2019). In dogs qPCR showed 100% specificity and a sensitivity higher than Baermann sedimentation, diagnosing several positive samples that were not revealed by Baermann possibly because qPCR also detected unviable larvae that could be missed at microscopy (Iatta et al., 2019). The authors suggested that coupling qPCR with Baermann could be an optimal approach to detect patent infections and reservoir dogs, although missed diagnoses could occur.

Studies suggest that positive PCR results in carnivore faecal samples decline significantly after 3 days from collection at room temperature (Santini et al., 2007). Long-term DNA preservation by cryopreservation or the use of chemical preservatives at room temperature (Beknazarova et al., 2017; Zhou et al., 2019) has been successfully employed, further discussion of which may be found in the *Pre-analytical variables in NAAT testing* section of this review.

7.4 Is *Strongyloides stercoralis* infection a zoonosis? From epidemiological evidence to haplotypes

To what extent strongyloidiasis is a zoonotic disease has been the subject of controversy in the literature for several decades, and what is the potential that dogs may serve as a source for human *S. stercoralis* infection, or vice versa, still remains a challenge.

Until 2017, the question of the identity of *S. stercoralis* from dogs and humans had not been thoroughly explored. Nine historical studies attempted to infect dogs with human strains from various parts of the world, but most infections were refractory or self-cured within weeks

(Galliard, 1951a; Fuelleborn, 1927; Sandground, 1928; Sandosham, 1952). A human isolate from Vietnam did cause lasting infection in a dog (Galliard, 1951b) and another from the Burma/Thailand region caused infection lasting 15 months in an immunosuppressed dog (Grove and Northern, 1982). The single published attempt to infect a human with a dog strain in the United States failed (Augustine and Davey, 1939).

There remains only one apparently confirmed transmission of *S. stercoralis* from dogs to a human documented in the scientific literature (Georgi and Sprinkle, 1974). In this case, the infected person demonstrated marked clinical symptoms (vomiting, abdominal pain and diarrhoea) and mounted an unusually high eosinophil response (13.6×10^9 cells/L), suggesting poor adaptation of the parasite to the human host. An unexplained case of autochthonous *S. stercoralis* infection in a girl from the United Kingdom raised the question of potential transmission from dog faeces while walking barefoot in parks (Sprott et al., 1987). Studies in the Anami Islands of Japan found no relationship between *Strongyloides* infection in dogs and their owners, despite a relatively high prevalence in each (10% and 2.8%, respectively) (Takano et al., 2009). Although zoonotic transmission from dogs is speculated and may be a phenomenon dependent upon the geographical origin of strains (Barratt and Sapp, 2020), it remains unclear why more infections in household contacts of infected dogs are not reported.

Attempts to distinguish *S. stercoralis* isolates from dogs and humans by means of molecular analysis and genotyping gave contradictory results against (Ramachandran et al., 1997; Hasegawa et al., 2009, 2010) or in support of (Schär et al., 2014) the zoonotic potential.

In 2017, two studies collecting samples from different geographical areas of Asia demonstrated that two distinct *cox1* clades of *S. stercoralis* exist, one found in both humans and dogs and the other restricted to dogs (Jaleta et al., 2017; Nagayasu et al., 2017). This demonstrated that dogs carry *S. stercoralis* genotypically indistinguishable from humans and non-human primates (NHPs) at the targets sequenced in addition to a dog specific population. The human/dog clade was associated with a single haplotype of HVR-IV (*cox1* lineage A), the other clade (dog only) had a unique HVR-IV haplotype (*cox1* lineage B). In dogs, the HVR IV haplotype may apparently be used to distinguish the two populations of *S. stercoralis* (Aupalee et al., 2020; Jaleta et al., 2017).

Beknazarova et al. (Beknazarova et al., 2019) found lineage A in both dogs and humans and lineage B affecting some dogs only in remote Australian communities. A limitation of this study, which incorporated deep sequencing of genotyping amplicons directly from faeces was that no control for coprophagia of human faeces by dogs was included. This is common activity for dogs in areas with poor sanitation and at least some of the genotypes identified may have been passage of *Strongyloides* DNA or larvae following consumption of human or animal faeces (Beknazarova et al., 2019). Interestingly, in further sequencing studies the parasites isolated from dogs from Thailand (Sanpool et al., 2019), Europe (Basso et al., 2019; Barratt et al., 2019), USA (Barratt et al., 2019) and Japan (Ko et al., 2020) belonged to the human/dog infective type (lineage A). A novel HVR-IV haplotype (haplotype E) has been identified in humans in China (Zhou et al., 2019) and from an Australian dog (Beknazarova et al., 2019).

It is now accepted that dogs can carry strains of *S. stercoralis* genetically very similar to those affecting humans, in addition to a dog-specific population (Beknazarova et al., 2019; Jaleta et al., 2017; Nagayasu et al., 2017). Although these studies provided support for zoonotic transmission, they cannot demonstrate that a direct transmission from dogs to humans occurs. A Barrat and Sapp (Barratt and Sapp, 2020) analysis recently suggested that some canine infections could represent incidental infections with strains originating from humans resulting in transient infection. The role of the cat as reservoir of infection is unexplored. Only one *S. stercoralis* isolate from a cat has been sequenced at *cox1* and was within the human/dog/NHP infecting lineage A (Wulcan et al., 2019).

It should be noted that the short length and limited discrimination of currently used genotyping targets disallows true phylogenetic comparison and longer more discriminatory targets must be identified before the question of zoonotic transmission can be finally settled (Bradbury et al., 2021b). The true role of domestic animals, specifically dogs (and cats) in the transmission and maintenance of *S. stercoralis* infections of humans remains unclear (Beknazarova et al., 2019; Barratt and Sapp, 2020; Bradbury et al., 2021b).

It has been demonstrated that *S. stercoralis* free-living cycle has only one generation and does not indefinitely persist in the environment as incorrectly perceived in the past, thus there is not an ongoing source of infection in the soil (Page et al., 2018). Although the most important reservoir of infection still remains people, the control of environmental reservoirs throughout sanitation and dog treatment may be required as part of the control strategies to break the life cycle of the parasite (Beknazarova et al., 2017; Page et al., 2018; Thamsborg et al., 2017). The WHO recently included the control of strongyloidiasis among the 2030 targets (Montresor et al., 2020). To reach this aim, the development of long read sequencing for *S. stercoralis* to definitively determine if dogs, or cats, act as reservoirs of human infection is of paramount importance (Bradbury et al., 2021b).

8. Systematic reviews with meta-analysis on diagnostic tests for human strongyloidiasis

Through the electronic search described in the methods, we identified three systematic reviews with meta-analysis evaluating diagnostic methods for human strongyloidiasis: one comparing coproparasitological techniques (Campo Polanco et al., 2014), one on serology (Kalantari et al., 2020), and one on molecular methods (Buonfrate et al., 2018b).

Main characteristics and findings of the reviews are summarized in Table 7.

From the results of these reviews, APC would appear to be the method with the highest sensitivity, but again the wide differences in the procedures applied for the same assay (e.g. number of plates cultured in APC, different DNA extraction methods for PCR), in the characteristics of the diagnostic assays themselves (e.g. different antigens used for serology assays), and in the reference tests for the estimation of accuracy hamper the comparison of methods and obtaining a definitive result.

9. The choice of a diagnostic test based on purpose and setting

Finally, the choice of diagnostic technique(s) to be implemented and the intensity of the diagnostic effort must be guided by the final aim of the investigation and the trade-off balance between easiness/implementability of the diagnostic procedure, consequences of inaccurate diagnosis and cost-effectiveness of treatment.

- In a context of initial epidemiological mapping of infection distribution, likely followed by preventive chemotherapy with ivermectin, extreme accuracy of the diagnosis at individual level is not required, since the estimates of prevalence would be used to evaluate a possible intervention with ivermectin at population level, and not an individual administration based on diagnosis on a single person (Buonfrate et al., 2021c). In this scenario, serology assays based on widely available techniques such as ELISA, prioritizing sensitivity and ease of use, might be currently the best option, also considering the possible collection of blood spots on filter paper (Formenti et al., 2016; Mounsey et al., 2014). However, accurate evaluation of cross-reactivity of assays is needed. In the same epidemiology investigation setting, but in the context of monitoring and evaluation of a control program, especially when infection prevalence falls, false positive results become a more important problem, and increased diagnostic effort towards specificity should be implemented (e.g. with the use of specific coproparasitological techniques directed at the retrieval of larvae, molecular techniques, or the two combined). In order to compare baseline and follow-up prevalence, it has been suggested that both serology and a faecal-based test would be used for baseline assessment, so that any of the two methods can be used in different phases of monitoring (depending on prevalence thresholds) (WHO, 2020).

- Especially outside the clinical context, the acceptability by the target population should also be considered for the choice of a test. Moreover, feasibility should be evaluated in terms of costs, technical skills (laboratory staff who can differentiate larvae for instance), logistics (such as transport of samples to referral laboratories), facilities and equipment (maintenance of cold chain, presence of equipment for molecular biology, etc.). Outside endemic areas, screening of populations with high epidemiological risk (such as migrants from endemic countries) should be based on a sensitive diagnostic tool (i.e. serology) (Requena-Méndez et al., 2017). A stool test is not mandatory; however, it will provide an indication of larval burden and in heavy infections may be useful to monitor treatment efficacy. Considering the possible harm of the infection against the high tolerability profile of ivermectin, treatment of all seropositive cases would be recommended (Requena-Méndez et al., 2017).
- For individual diagnosis in people with suspected infection (including those at risk of developing hyperinfection/disseminated infection, such as candidates to immunosuppressant treatments) a combination of serology with a sensitive faecal test (which could be parasitological or molecular, depending on the expertise/equipment of the laboratory) would be suggested, in order to further increase sensitivity and to monitor treatment response (Requena-Méndez et al., 2017).
- In immunocompromised people, serology might be negative (Abdul-Fattah et al., 1995; Ahmed et al., 2019). However, the combination of serology with a sensitive faecal test would be still recommended.
- Finally, in the context of a clinical trial of drugs efficacy, particular care must be taken to use a sensitive faecal test, which should be better repeated over time in the follow-up phase, to safely rule out the persistence of the infection (Sato et al., 1995; Dreyer et al., 1996). In non-endemic areas, clinical trials relying on serologic follow-up have also been conducted (Bisoffi et al., 2011). In this case, time-point(s) for follow-up should be at least 5–6 months after treatment, in order to observe either a seroconversion or a decline in titre (Biggs et al., 2009; Buonfrate et al., 2015; Loutfy et al., 2002; Page et al., 2006; Ramanathan et al., 2008). Because of the high risk of re-infection during a long-term follow up, serology would not be adequate for clinical trials in endemic area.

A summary of these points is presented in Table 6.

Table 6 Diagnostic test recommendation based on setting and purpose.

Population-based testing		Serological tests	Stool conventional/ molecular tests[a]	Notes
Endemic Areas	Epidemiological Mapping	+	(+)	Ease of use and acceptability of serology
				Sub-population for stool-based testing for quality assurance and baseline data
	Evaluation of Control Program efficacy	(+)	(+)	Test a sub-population include stool testing (delayed sero-reversion/re-infection)
Non-endemic Areas	General screening of populations with risk factors (e.g. refugee health clinics)	+	(+)	Ease of use of serology
				Consider stool testing seropositive to determine disease burden/follow treatment efficacy
Individual Testing[b]				
Risk factor based	Immunocompromise (pre-treatment or existing)	+	+	Serology sensitivity decreased Maximize diagnostic potential where possible
	Symptomatic/Clinical Indication	+	+	Use available tests
Clinical Trial	Drug Therapy	(+)	+	Stool testing for clearance preferred
				Sero-reversion in non-endemic areas

[a]Conventional and/or molecular stool test based on availability/feasibility.
[b]Endemic or non-endemic areas.

Table 7 Main characteristics and findings of systematic reviews estimating the accuracy of different diagnostic tests.

Study	Reference test(s) used in the included papers	Diagnostic methods evaluated	Sensitivity (95%CI); specificity (95% CI)	Notes
Campo Polanco et al. (2014)	Combination of the results of all parasitological tests applied on the panel of stool	1. Stool microscopy without concentration	Se 21% (16–26); Sp 100%	
		2. Formol-ether concentration stool microscopy	Se 48% (42–54); Sp100%	
		3. Baermann method	Se 72% (67–76); Sp100%	
		4. Agar plate culture	Se 89% (86–92); Sp100%	
Kalantari et al. (2020)	Faecal-based techniques, including culture, Baermann, DS, FECT, Kato-Katz	Serology (IFAT and ELISA)	Se 71.7% (56–83.4); Sp 90% (81–95)	Different sensitivity depending on the *Strongyloides* species used as antigenic preparation: from 81% (60–92) with *S. venezuelenzis* to 49% (23–74) with *S. ratti*
Buonfrate et al. (2018b)	Coproparasitological methods only	PCR (conventional, nested and real-time)	Se 71.8% (52.3–85.5); Sp 93.5% (90.3–95.6)	For real-time PCR: 56.5% (39.2–72.4) and 95.4% (91.7–97.5) against combination of methods and 64.4% (46.2–77.7) and 64.4% (46.2–77.7) against parasitological methods only
	A combination of coproparasitological and serological methods	PCR (conventional, nested and real-time)	Se 61.8% (42–78.4); Sp 95.3% (92–97.2)	

10. Conclusions

With this review, we have attempted to outline, as accurately and completely as possible, the state of the art and future perspectives for the diagnosis of *S. stercoralis*, a parasite with unique characteristics. While traditional faecal methods, which use microscopic identification, have a high specificity in the hands of trained operators, the reduced sensitivity of these methods, due to variable larval output and pre-analytical limitations, has been the main cause of the underestimation of the prevalence of this helminth and consequently of its importance for public health. Routine clinical diagnosis is affected by the limitations of diagnostic tests, and it is important to consider the diagnosis when there are epidemiological risk factors. In addition, research studies can be impacted by diagnostic limitations as the infection may be present, even in apparently uninfected control groups.

However, significant progress has been made and is ongoing, with many different and new diagnostic techniques available and others being implemented. The challenge faced now is to determine the most appropriate diagnostics or combination of diagnostics for different purposes, the most immediate being the assessment of the burden of infection and disease in endemic countries and monitoring of progress towards the ambitious goals set by the WHO for 2030.

References

Abdul-Fattah, M.M., Nasr, M.E., Yousef, S.M., Ibraheem, M.I., Abdul-Wahhab, S.E., Soliman, H.M., 1995. Efficacy of ELISA in diagnosis of strongyloidiasis among the immune-compromised patients. J. Egypt. Soc. Parasitol. 25, 491–498.

Ahmad, H., Balachandra, D., Arifin, N., Nolan, T.J., Lok, J.B., Hayat Khan, A., Yunus, M.H., Noordin, R., 2020. Diagnostic potential of an IgE-ELISA in detecting strongyloidiasis. Am. J. Trop. Med. Hyg. 103, 2288–2293.

Ahmadi, N.A., Damraj, F.-A., 2009. A field evaluation of formalin-gasoline technique in the concentration of stool for detection of intestinal parasites. Parasitol. Res. 104, 553–557.

Ahmadi, N.A., Pakdad, K., 2007. Tween as a substitute for diethyl ether in the formalin-ether sedimentation technique. Iran. J. Public Health 36, 91–95.

Ahmed, S.A., EL-Moselhy, A., EL-Moammaly, A., EL-Shewy, K., 2019. Strongyloides stercoralis in patients on corticosteroids therapy using enzyme-linked immunosorbent assay and gelatin particles indirect agglutination tests: A diagnostic approach. Acta Parasitologica 64, 394–405.

Albonico, M., Becker, S.L., Odermatt, P., Angheben, A., Anselmi, M., Amor, A., Barda, B., Buonfrate, D., Cooper, P., Gétaz, L., Keiser, J., Khieu, V., Montresor, A., Muñoz, J., Requena-Méndez, A., Savioli, L., Speare, R., Steinmann, P., van Lieshout, L., Utzinger, J., Bisoffi, Z., 2016. StrongNet: an international network to improve diagnostics and access to treatment for strongyloidiasis control. PLoS Negl. Trop. Dis. 10, e0004898.

Allen, A.V., Ridley, D.S., 1970. Further observations on the formol-ether concentration technique for faecal parasites. J. Clin. Pathol. 23, 545–546.

Amor, A., Rodriguez, E., Saugar, J.M., Arroyo, A., López-Quintana, B., Abera, B., Yimer, M., Yizengaw, E., Zewdie, D., Ayehubizu, Z., Hailu, T., Mulu, W., Echazú, A., Krolewieki, A.J., Aparicio, P., Herrador, Z., Anegagrie, M., Benito, A., 2016. High prevalence of Strongyloides stercoralis in school-aged children in a rural highland of North-Western Ethiopia: the role of intensive diagnostic work-up. Parasit. Vectors 9 (1), 617. https://doi.org/10.1186/s13071-016-1912-8. PMID: 27903301; PMCID: PMC5131444.

Anamnart, W., Pattanawongsa, A., Intapan, P.M., Maleewong, W., 2010. Factors affecting recovery of Strongyloides stercoralis larvae: an approach to a newly modified formalin-ether concentration technique for diagnosis of strongyloidiasis. J. Clin. Microbiol. 48, 97–100.

Anamnart, W., Intapan, P.M., Maleewong, W., 2013. Modified formalin-ether concentration technique for diagnosis of human strongyloidiasis. Korean J. Parasitol. 51, 743–745.

Anderson, N.W., Klein, D.M., Dornink, S.M., Jespersen, D.J., Kubofcik, J., Nutman, T.B., Merrigan, S.D., Couturier, M.R., Theel, E.S., 2014. Comparison of three immunoassays for detection of antibodies to Strongyloides stercoralis. Clin. Vaccine Immunol. 21, 732–736.

Andreetta Corral, M., de Paula, F.M., Meisel, D., Abdala, E., Figueiredo Costa, S., Camera Pierrotti, L., Yamashiro, J., do Nascimento Gonçalves, E.M., Castilho, V.L.P., Chieffi, P.P., Gryschek, R.C.B., 2019. IgG reactivity with 40-35 kDa soluble and membrane antigen of Strongyloides venezuelensis in immunocompromised patients. Acta Trop. 190, 357–360.

Anecimo, R.S., Tonani, K.A., Fregonesi, B.M., Mariano, A.P., Ferrassino, M.D., Trevilato, T.M., Rodrigues, R.B., Segura-Munoz, S.I., 2012. Adaptation of Ritchie's method for parasites diagnosing with minimization of chemical products. Interdiscip Perspect Infect Dis 2012, 409757.

Arakaki, T., Hasegawa, H., Asato, R., Ikeshiro, T., Kinjo, F., Saito, A., Iwanaga, M., 1988. A new method to detect Strongylides stercoralis from human stool. Japan J. Trop. Med. Hyg. 16, 11–17.

Arakaki, T., Iwanaga, M., Kinjo, F., Saito, A., Asato, R., Ikeshiro, T., 1990. Efficacy of agar-plate culture in detection of Strongyloides stercoralis infection. J. Parasitol. 76, 425–428.

Aramendia, A.A., Anegagrie, M., Zewdie, D., Dacal, E., Saugar, J.M., Herrador, Z., Hailu, T., Yimer, M., Periago, M.V., Rodriguez, E., Benito, A., 2020. Epidemiology of intestinal helminthiases in a rural community of Ethiopia: is it time to expand control programs to include strongyloides stercoralis and the entire community? PLoS Negl. Trop. Dis. 14, 1–14.

Arifin, N., Riazi, M., Mahmoud, S.S., Yunus, M.H., Low, H.C., Mohamed, Z., Noordin, R., 2013. Improvement of serodiagnosis of human strongyloidiasis. Trop. Med. Int. Health 18, 61.

Arifin, N., Hanafiah, K.M., Ahmad, H., Noordin, R., 2019. Serodiagnosis and early detection of Strongyloides stercoralis infection. *Journal of microbiology, immunology, and infection* =. Wei mian yu gan ran za zhi 52, 371–378.

Atkins, N.S., Lindo, J.F., Lee, M.G., Conway, D.J., Bailey, J.W., Robinson, R.D., Bundy, D.A., 1997. Humoral responses in human strongyloidiasis: correlations with infection chronicity. Trans. R. Soc. Trop. Med. Hyg. 91, 609–613.

Augustine, D., Davey, D., 1939. Observations on a natural infection with Strongyloides in the dog. J. Parasitol. Res. 25, 117–119.

Aupalee, K., Wijit, A., Singphai, K., Rödelsperger, C., Zhou, S., Saeung, A., Streit, A., 2020. Genomic studies on Strongyloides stercoralis in northern and western Thailand. Parasit. Vectors 13, 250.

Autier, B., Belaz, S., Razakandrainibe, R., Gangneux, J.P., Robert-Gangneux, F., 2018. Comparison of three commercial multiplex PCR assays for the diagnosis of intestinal protozoa. Parasite 25, 48.

Ayana, M., Cools, P., Mekonnen, Z., Biruksew, A., Dana, D., Rashwan, N., Prichard, R., Vlaminck, J., Verweij, J.J., Levecke, B., 2019. Comparison of four DNA extraction and three preservation protocols for the molecular detection and quantification of soil-transmitted helminths in stool. PLoS Negl. Trop. Dis. 13, e0007778.

Baermann, G., 1917. A Simple Method for the Detection of Ankylostomum (Nematde) Larvae in Soil Tests. Javasche Boekhandel & Drukkerij.

Balachandra, D., Ahmad, H., Arifin, N., Noordin, R., 2021. Direct detection of Strongyloides infection via molecular and antigen detection methods. Eur. J. Clin. Microbiol. Infect. Dis. 40, 27–37.

Barda, B., Wampfler, R., Sayasone, S., Phongluxa, K., Xayavong, S., Keoduangsy, K., Schindler, C., Keiser, J., 2018. Evaluation of two DNA extraction methods for detection of Strongyloides stercoralis infection. J. Clin. Microbiol. 56.

Barratt, J.L.N., Sapp, S.G.H., 2020. Machine learning-based analyses support the existence of species complexes for Strongyloides fuelleborni and Strongyloides stercoralis. Parasitology 147, 1184–1195.

Barratt, J.L.N., Lane, M., Talundzic, E., Richins, T., Robertson, G., Formenti, F., Pritt, B., Verocai, G., Nascimento de Souza, J., Mato Soares, N., Traub, R., Buonfrate, D., Bradbury, R.S., 2019. A global genotyping survey of Strongyloides stercoralis and Strongyloides fuelleborni using deep amplicon sequencing. PLoS Negl. Trop. Dis. 13, e0007609.

Barrett, J., Broderick, C., Soulsby, H., Wade, P., Newsholme, W., 2016. Subcutaneous ivermectin use in the treatment of severe Strongyloides stercoralis infection: two case reports and a discussion of the literature. J. Antimicrob. Chemother. 71, 220–225.

Basáñez, M.-G., Marshall, C., Carabin, H., Gyorkos, T., Joseph, L., 2004. Bayesian statistics for parasitologists. Trends Parasitol. 20, 85–91.

Basso, W., Grandt, L.-M., Magnenat, A.-L., Gottstein, B., Campos, M., 2019. Strongyloides stercoralis infection in imported and local dogs in Switzerland: from clinics to molecular genetics. Parasitol. Res. 118, 255–266.

Becker, S.L., Piraisoody, N., Kramme, S., Marti, H., Silué, K.D., Panning, M., Nickel, B., Kern, W.V., Herrmann, M., Hatz, C.F., N'Goran, E.K., Utzinger, J., von Müller, L., 2015. Real-time PCR for detection of Strongyloides stercoralis in human stool samples from Côte d'Ivoire: diagnostic accuracy, inter-laboratory comparison and patterns of hookworm co-infection. Acta Trop. 150, 210–217.

Beknazarova, M., Millsteed, S., Robertson, G., Whiley, H., Ross, K., 2017. Validation of DESS as a DNA preservation method for the detection of Strongyloides spp. in canine feces. Int. J. Environ. Res. Public Health 14.

Beknazarova, M., Barratt, J.L.N., Bradbury, R.S., Lane, M., Whiley, H., Ross, K., 2019. Detection of classic and cryptic Strongyloides genotypes by deep amplicon sequencing: A preliminary survey of dog and human specimens collected from remote Australian communities. PLoS Negl. Trop. Dis. 13, e0007241.

Beknazarova, M., Whiley, H., Traub, R., Ross, K., 2020. Opportunistic mapping of Strongyloides stercoralis and hookworm in dogs in remote Australian communities. Pathogens (Basel, Switzerland) 9.

Benjamin-Chung, J., Crider, Y., Mertens, A., Ercumen, A., Pickering, A., Lin, A., Steinbaum, L., Swarthout, J., Rahman, M., Parvez, S., Haque, R., Njenga, S., Kihara, J., Null, C., Luby, S., Colford, J., Arnold, B., 2021. Household finished flooring and soil-transmitted helminth and giardia infections among children in rural Bangladesh and Kenya: a prospective cohort study. Lancet Glob. Health 9, e301–e308.

Biggs, B.-A., Caruana, S., Mihrshahi, S., Jolley, D., Leydon, J., Chea, L., Nuon, S., 2009. Management of chronic strongyloidiasis in immigrants and refugees: is serologic testing useful? Am. J. Trop. Med. Hyg. 80, 788–791.
Bisoffi, Z., Buonfrate, D., Angheben, A., Boscolo, M., Anselmi, M., Marocco, S., Monteiro, G., Gobbo, M., Bisoffi, G., Gobbi, F., 2011. Randomized clinical trial on ivermectin versus thiabendazole for the treatment of strongyloidiasis. PLoS Negl. Trop. Dis. 5, e1254.
Bisoffi, Z., Buonfrate, D., Sequi, M., Mejia, R., Cimino, R.O., Krolewiecki, A.J., Albonico, M., Gobbo, M., Bonafini, S., Angheben, A., Requena-Mendez, A., Muñoz, J., Nutman, T.B., 2014. Diagnostic accuracy of five serologic tests for Strongyloides stercoralis infection. PLoS Negl. Trop. Dis. 8, e2640.
Black, M.A., Craig, B.A., 2002. Estimating disease prevalence in the absence of a gold standard. Stat. Med. 21, 2653–2669.
Blatt, J.M., Cantos, G.A., 2003. Evaluation of techniques for the diagnosis of Strongyloides stercoralis in human immunodeficiency virus (HIV) positive and HIV negative individuals in the city of Itajaí. Brazil. Braz. J. Infect. Dis 7, 402–408.
Blotkamp, J., Krepel, H.P., Kumar, V., Baeta, S., Van'T Noordende, J.M., Polderman, A.M., 1993. Observations on the morphology of adults and larval stages of Oesophagostomum sp. isolated from man in northern Togo and Ghana. J. Helminthol. 67, 49–61.
Bon, B., Houze, S., Talabani, H., Magne, D., Belkadi, G., Develoux, M., Senghor, Y., Chandenier, J., Ancelle, T., Hennequin, C., 2010. Evaluation of a rapid enzyme-linked immunosorbent assay for diagnosis of strongyloidiasis. J. Clin. Microbiol. 48, 1716–1719.
Boscolo, M., Gobbo, M., Mantovani, W., Degani, M., Anselmi, M., Monteiro, G.B., Marocco, S., Angheben, A., Mistretta, M., Santacatterina, M., Tais, S., Bisoffi, Z., 2007. Evaluation of an indirect immunofluorescence assay for strongyloidiasis as a tool for diagnosis and follow-up. Clin. Vaccine Immunol. 14, 129–133.
Bosqui, L.R., Gonçalves, A.L.R., Gonçalves-Pires, M.D.R.F., Custodio, L.A., de Menezes, M.C.N.D., Murad, V.A., de Paula, F.M., Pavanelli, W.R., Conchon-Costa, I., Costa-Cruz, J.M., Costa, I.N., 2015. Detection of parasite-specific IgG and IgA in paired serum and saliva samples for diagnosis of human strongyloidiasis in northern Paraná state, Brazil. Acta Trop. 150, 190–195.
Bosqui, L.R., Gonzaga, H.T., Gonçalves-Pires, M.D.R.D.F., de Paula, F.M., Almeida, R.S., Pavanelli, W.R., Conchon-Costa, I., Costa-Cruz, J.M., da Costa, I.N., 2017. Avidity as a criterion for diagnosis of human strongyloidiasis increases specificity of IgG ELISA. Diagn. Microbiol. Infect. Dis. 89, 262–264.
Bradbury, R.S., 2019. Ternidens deminutus revisited: A review of human infections with the false hookworm. *Trop med.* Infect. Dis. 4.
Bradbury, R., 2021. Strongyloides fuelleborni kellyi in New Guinea: neglected, ignored and unexplored. Microbiol. Aust. 42, 169–172.
Bradbury, R., Herwaldt, B.L., 2020. Section VIII-C: parasitic agents. In: Potts, P.J.M.J. (Ed.), Biosafety in Microbiological and Biomedical Laboratories. National library of Medine, Washington DC.
Bradbury, R.S., Arguello, I., Lane, M., Cooley, G., Handali, S., Dimitrova, S.D., Nascimento, F.S., Jameson, S., Hellmann, K., Tharp, M., Byers, P., Montgomery, S.P., Haynie, L., Kirmse, B., Pilotte, N., Williams, S.A., Hobbs, C.V., 2020. Parasitic infection surveillance in Mississippi Delta children. Am. J. Trop. Med. Hyg. 103, 1150–1153.
Bradbury, R.S., Lane, M., Arguello, I., Handali, S., Cooley, G., Pilotte, N., Williams, J.M., Jameson, S., Montgomery, S.P., Hellmann, K., Tharp, M., Haynie, L., Galloway, R., Brackin, B., Kirmse, B., Stempak, L., Byers, P., Williams, S., Faruque, F., Hobbs, C.V., 2021a. Parasitic disease surveillance, Mississippi, USA. Emerg. Infect. Dis. 27, 2201–2204.

Bradbury, R.S., Pafčo, B., Nosková, E., Hasegawa, H., 2021b. Strongyloides genotyping: a review of methods and application in public health and population genetics. Int. J. Parasitol. 51, 1153–1166.

Brasil, R., Badaró, R., Andrade, J.A.F.D., Andrade, T.M.D., Carvalho, E.M., 1988. Diagnóstico sorológico da estrongiloidíase humana, através do método imunoenzimático TT - Immunoenzymatic serological diagnosis of human strongyloidiasis. Rev. Soc. Bras. Med. Trop. 21, 139–143.

Buonfrate, D., Requena-Mendez, A., Angheben, A., Muñoz, J., Gobbi, F., van Den Ende, J., Bisoffi, Z., 2013. Severe strongyloidiasis: a systematic review of case reports. BMC Infect. Dis. 13, 78.

Buonfrate, D., Sequi, M., Mejia, R., Cimino, R.O., Krolewiecki, A.J., Albonico, M., Degani, M., Tais, S., Angheben, A., Requena-Mendez, A., Muñoz, J., Nutman, T.B., Bisoffi, Z., 2015. Accuracy of five serologic tests for the follow up of Strongyloides stercoralis infection. PLoS Negl. Trop. Dis. 9, e0003491.

Buonfrate, D., Paradies, P., Iarussi, F., Formenti, F., Perandin, F., Otranto, D., Bisoffi, Z., 2017a. Serological and molecular tests for the diagnosis of Strongyloides stercoralis infection in dogs. Parasitol. Res. 116, 2027–2029.

Buonfrate, D., Perandin, F., Formenti, F., Bisoffi, Z., 2017b. A retrospective study comparing agar plate culture, indirect immunofluorescence and real-time PCR for the diagnosis of Strongyloides stercoralis infection. Parasitology 144, 812–816.

Buonfrate, D., Gobbi, F., Angheben, A., Bisoffi, Z., 2018a. Strongyloides stercoralis: the need for accurate information. Lancet 391, 2322–2323.

Buonfrate, D., Requena-Mendez, A., Angheben, A., Cinquini, M., Cruciani, M., Fittipaldo, A., Giorli, G., Gobbi, F., Piubelli, C., Bisoffi, Z., 2018b. Accuracy of molecular biology techniques for the diagnosis of Strongyloides stercoralis infection-A systematic review and meta-analysis. PLoS Negl. Trop. Dis. 12, e0006229.

Buonfrate, D., Salas-Coronas, J., Muñoz, J., Maruri, B.T., Rodari, P., Castelli, F., Zammarchi, L., Bianchi, L., Gobbi, F., Cabezas-Fernández, T., Requena-Mendez, A., Godbole, G., Silva, R., Romero, M., Chiodini, P.L., Bisoffi, Z., 2019. Multiple-dose versus single-dose ivermectin for Strongyloides stercoralis infection (strong treat 1 to 4): a multicentre, open-label, phase 3, randomised controlled superiority trial. Lancet Infect. Dis. 19, 1181–1190.

Buonfrate, D., Bisanzio, D., Giorli, G., Odermatt, P., Fürst, T., Greenaway, C., French, M., Reithinger, R., Gobbi, F., Montresor, A., Bisoffi, Z., 2020. The global prevalence of Strongyloides stercoralis infection. Pathogens 9.

Buonfrate, D., Fittipaldo, A., Vlieghe, E., Bottieau, E., 2021a. Clinical and laboratory features of Strongyloides stercoralis infection at diagnosis and after treatment: a systematic review and meta-analysis. Clin. Microbiol. Infect. 27, 1621–1628.

Buonfrate, D., Marrone, R., Silva, R., Mirisola, C., Ragusa, A., Mistretta, M., Perandin, F., Bisoffi, Z., 2021b. Prevalence of strongyloidiasis in a cohort of migrants in Italy and accuracy of a novel ELISA assay for S. stercoralis infection, a cross-sectional study. Microorganisms 9.

Buonfrate, D., Zammarchi, L., Bisoffi, Z., Montresor, A., Boccalini, S., 2021c. Control programs for strongyloidiasis in areas of high endemicity: an economic analysis of different approaches. Infect. Dis. Poverty 10, 76.

Campo Polanco, L., Gutiérrez, L.A., Cardona Arias, J., 2014. Diagnosis of Strongyloides Stercoralis infection: meta-analysis on evaluation of conventional parasitological methods (1980-2013). Rev. Esp. Salud Publica 88, 581–600.

Campo-Polanco, L.F., Sarmiento, J.M.H., Mesa, M.A., Franco, C.J.V., López, L., Botero, L.E., Builes, L.A.G., 2018. Strongyloidiasis in humans: diagnostic efficacy of four conventional methods and real-time polymerase chain reaction. Rev. Soc. Bras. Med. Trop. 51, 493–502.

Carvalho, G.L.X.D., Moreira, L.E., Pena, J.L., Marinho, C.C., Bahia, M.T., Machado-Coelho, G.L.L., 2012. A comparative study of the TF-test®, Kato-Katz, Hoffman-Pons-Janer, Willis and Baermann-Moraes coprologic methods for the detection of human parasitosis. Mem. Inst. Oswaldo Cruz 107, 80–84.
Cervone, M., Giannelli, A., Otranto, D., Perrucci, S., 2016. Strongyloides stercoralis hyperinfection in an immunosuppressed dog from France. Rev. Veterinaire Clin. 51, 55–59.
Chankongsin, S., Wampfler, R., Ruf, M.T., Odermatt, P., Marti, H., Nickel, B., Keoluangkhot, V., Neumayr, A., 2020. Strongyloides stercoralis prevalence and diagnostics in Vientiane, Lao People's Democratic Republic. Infect. Dis. Poverty 9, 133.
Chaves, L.A., Gonçalves, A.L.R., Paula, F.M., Silva, N.M., Silva, C.V., Costa-Cruz, J.M., Freitas, M.A.R., 2015. Comparison of parasitological, immunological and molecular methods for evaluation of fecal samples of immunosuppressed rats experimentally infected with Strongyloides venezuelensis. Parasitology 142, 1715–1721.
Cohen, J.F., KorevaaR, D.A., Altman, D.G., Bruns, D.E., Gatsonis, C.A., Hooft, L., Irwig, L., Levine, D., Reitsma, J.B., De Vet, H.C., Bossuyt, P.M., 2016. STARD 2015 guidelines for reporting diagnostic accuracy studies: explanation and elaboration. BMJ Open 6, e012799.
Conway, D.J., Bailey, J.W., Lindo, J.F., Robinson, R.D., Bundy, D.A., Bianco, A.E., 1993. Serum IgG reactivity with 41-, 31-, and 28-kDa larval proteins of Strongyloides stercoralis in individuals with strongyloidiasis. J Infect Dis 168, 784–787.
Cools, P., Vlaminck, J., Albonico, M., Ame, S., Ayana, M., José Antonio, B.P., Cringoli, G., Dana, D., Keiser, J., Maurelli, M.P., Maya, C., Matoso, L.F., Montresor, A., Mekonnen, Z., Mirams, G., Corrêa-Oliveira, R., Pinto, S.A., Rinaldi, L., Sayasone, S., Thomas, E., Verweij, J.J., Vercruysse, J., Levecke, B., 2019. Diagnostic performance of a single and duplicate Kato-Katz, mini-FLOTAC, FECPAKG2 and qPCR for the detection and quantification of soil-transmitted helminths in three endemic countries. PLoS Negl. Trop. Dis. 13, e0007446.
Corral, M.A., Paula, F.M., Gottardi, M., Meisel, D.M.C.L., Chieffi, P.P., Gryschek, R.C.B., 2015. Membrane fractions from Strongyloides venezuelensis in the immunodiagnosis of human strongyloidiasis TT - Frações de membrana de Strongyloides venezuelensis para o imunodiagnóstico da estrongiloidíase humana. Rev. Inst. Med. Trop. Säo Paulo 57, 77–80.
Costa-Cruz, J.M., Bullamah, C.B., Gonçalves-Pires, M.D.R., Campos, D.M., Vieira, M.A., 1997. Cryo-microtome sections of coproculture larvae of Strongyloides stercoralis and Strongyloides ratti as antigen sources for the immunodiagnosis of human strongyloidiasis. Rev. Inst. Med. Trop. Sao Paulo 39, 313–317.
Coutinho, J., Campos, R., Amato Neto, V., 1951. Nota sobre o diagnostico e prevalencia de estrongiloidose em Sao Paulo. Rev. Clin. Sao Paulo 27, 11–20.
Cringoli, G., Rinaldi, L., Maurelli, M.P., Utzinger, J., 2010. FLOTAC: new multivalent techniques for qualitative and quantitative copromicroscopic diagnosis of parasites in animals and humans. Nat. Protoc. 5, 503–515.
Cringoli, G., Rinaldi, L., Albonico, M., Bergquist, R., Utzinger, J., 2013. Geospatial (s)tools: integration of advanced epidemiological sampling and novel diagnostics. Geospat. Health 7, 399–404.
Cvetkovikj, A., Rashikj, L., Celeska, I., Petrov, E., 2018. First case of Strongyloides Stercoralis infection in a dog in the republic of Macedonia. Maced. Vet. Rev. 41, 95–98.
Dacal, E., Saugar, J.M., Soler, T., Azcárate, J.M., Jiménez, M.S., Merino, F.J., Rodríguez, E., 2018. Parasitological versus molecular diagnosis of strongyloidiasis in serial stool samples: how many? J. Helminthol. 92, 12–16.
Dancescu, P., 1968. Investigations on the intensity of the infection in a strongyloidiasis focus. The coal culture method. Trans. R. Soc. Trop. Med. Hyg. 62, 490–495.

Dashchenko, S., Soroka, N., Semenko, O., 2020. Distribution of Strongyloides Stercoralis among dogs of different housing groups in KYIV and KYIV region. Clinical Manifestations And Diagnostic Methods. *EUREKA: Health Sciences* 5, 99–107.

de Kaminsky, R.G., 1993. Evaluation of three methods for laboratory diagnosis of Strongyloides stercoralis infection. J. Parasitol. 79, 277–280.

de Souza, J.N., Langford, I.I., Wang, Y., Soares, N.M., Handali, S., 2021. Development of rSs-NIE-1 and rSs-IR recombinant antigen-based immunoblot for detection of antibody to Strongyloides stercoralis. Am. J. Trop. Med. Hyg. 104, 2038–2041.

Dendukuri, N., Joseph, L., 2001. Bayesian approaches to modeling the conditional dependence between multiple diagnostic tests. Biometrics 57, 158–167.

Dendukuri, N., Bélisle, P., Joseph, L., 2010. Bayesian sample size for diagnostic test studies in the absence of a gold standard: comparing identifiable with non-identifiable models. Stat. Med. 29, 2688–2697.

Dillard, K.J., Saari, S.A., Anttila, M., 2007. Strongyloides stercoralis infection in a Finnish kennel. Acta Vet. Scand. 49, 37.

Dreyer, G., Fernandes-Silva, E., Alves, S., Rocha, A., Albuquerque, R., Addiss, D., 1996. Patterns of detection of Strongyloides stercoralis in stool specimens: implications for diagnosis and clinical trials. J. Clin. Microbiol. 34, 2569–2571.

Eamudomkarn, C., Sithithaworn, P., Sithithaworn, J., Kaewkes, S., Sripa, B., Itoh, M., 2015. Comparative evaluation of Strongyloides ratti and S. stercoralis larval antigen for diagnosis of strongyloidiasis in an endemic area of opisthorchiasis. Parasitol. Res. 114, 2543–2551.

Erdman, D.D., 1981. Clinical comparison of ethyl acetate and diethyl ether in the formalin-ether sedimentation technique. J. Clin. Microbiol. 14, 483–485.

Eydal, M., Skirnisson, K., 2016. Strongyloides stercoralis found in imported dogs, household dogs and kennel dogs in Iceland. Icel Agric Sci. 29, 39–51.

Faust, E., D'antonio, J., Odon, V., Miller, M., Perez, C., Sawitz, W., Thomen, F., Tobie, J., Walker, H., 1938. A critical study of clinical laboratory technics for the diagnosis of protozoan cysts and helminth eggs in feces. Am. J. Trop. Med. Hyg. 18, 169–183.

Faust, E.C., Sawitz, W., Tobie, J., Odon, V., Peres, C., Linicome, D., 1939. Comparative efficiency of various technics for the diagnosis of protozoa and helminths in feces. J. Parasitol. 25, 241–262.

Feliciano, N.D., Ribeiro, V.D.S., Santos, F.D.A.A., Fujimura, P.T., Gonzaga, H.T., Goulart, L.R., Costa-Cruz, J.M., 2014. Bacteriophage-fused peptides for serodiagnosis of human strongyloidiasis. PLoS Negl. Trop. Dis. 8, e2792.

Fernández-Soto, P., Sánchez-Hernández, A., Gandasegui, J., Bajo Santos, C., López-Abán, J., Saugar, J.M., Rodríguez, E., Vicente, B., Muro, A., 2016. Strong-LAMP: A LAMP assay for Strongyloides spp. detection in stool and urine samples. Towards the diagnosis of human strongyloidiasis starting from a rodent model. PLoS Negl. Trop. Dis. 10, e0004836.

Fernández-Soto, P., Celis-Giraldo, C.T., Collar-Fernández, C., Gorgojo, Ó., Camargo, M., Muñoz, J., Salas-Coronas, J., Patarroyo, M.A., Muro, A., 2020. Strong-LAMP assay based on a Strongyloides spp.-derived partial sequence in the 18S rRNA as potential biomarker for strongyloidiasis diagnosis in human urine samples. Dis. Markers 2020 (5265198).

Formenti, F., Buonfrate, D., Prandi, R., Marquez, M., Caicedo, C., Rizzi, E., Guevara, A.G., Vicuña, Y., Huerlo, F.R., Perandin, F., Bisoffi, Z., Anselmi, M., 2016. Comparison of S. stercoralis serology performed on dried blood spots and on conventional serum samples. Front. Microbiol. 7, 1778.

Formenti, F., La Marca, G., Perandin, F., Pajola, B., Romano, M., Santucci, B., Silva, R., Giorli, G., Bisoffi, Z., Buonfrate, D., 2019. A diagnostic study comparing conventional and real-time PCR for Strongyloides stercoralis on urine and on faecal samples. Acta Trop. 190, 284–287.

Fradejas, I., Herrero-Martínez, J.M., Lizasoaín, M., De Las, R., Parras, E., Pérez-Ayala, A., 2018. Comparative study of two commercial tests for Strongyloides stercoralis serologic diagnosis. Trans. R. Soc. Trop. Med. Hyg. 112, 561–567.

Fuelleborn, F., 1927. Über das Verhalten der Larven von Strongyloides Stercoralis, Hakenwürmern und Ascaris lumbricoides im Körper des Wirtes. *Arch. Schiffs.-u.* Tropenhyg 31, 1–56.

Galliard, H., 1951a. Experimental infestation with Strongyloides stercoralis in Tonkin; part 2. Ann. Parasitol. Hum. Comp. 26, 67–84.

Galliard, H., 1951b. Study on the experimental infestation with Strongyloides stercoralis in Tonkin. XII. Action of physical and chemical factors on the endogenous and exogenous development. Ann. Parasitol. Hum. Comp. 26, 201–227.

Garrett, P., Lasky, F., Meier, K., 2008. User protocol for evaluation of qualitative test performance; approved guideline, second ed. Clinical and Laboratory Standards Institute, Wayne, PA.

Gelaye, W., Williams, N.A., Kepha, S., Junior, A.M., Fleitas, P.E., Marti-Soler, H., Damtie, D., Menkir, S., Krolewiecki, A.J., Van Lieshout, L., Enbiale, W., 2021. Performance evaluation of Baermann techniques: the quest for developing a microscopy reference standard for the diagnosis of Strongyloides stercoralis. PLoS Negl. Trop. Dis. 15, e0009076.

Georgi, J.R., Sprinkle, C.L., 1974. A case of human strongyloidosis apparently contracted from asymptomatic colony dogs. Am. J. Trop. Med. Hyg. 23, 899–901.

Getaneh, A., Medhin, G., Shimelis, T., 2010. Cryptosporidium and Strongyloides stercoralis infections among people with and without HIV infection and efficiency of diagnostic methods for Strongyloides in Yirgalem hospital, southern Ethiopia. BMC. Res. Notes 3, 90.

Ghasemikhah, R., Tabatabaiefar, M.A., Shariatzadeh, S.A., Shahbazi, A., Hazratian, T., 2017. A PCR-Based Molecular Detection of Strongyloides Stercoralisin Human Stool Samples from Tabriz City. Scientia pharmaceutica, Iran, p. 85.

Glinz, D., Silué, K.D., Knopp, S., Lohourignon, L.K., Yao, K.P., Steinmann, P., Rinaldi, L., Cringoli, G., N'goran, E. K. & Utzinger, J., 2010. Comparing diagnostic accuracy of Kato-Katz, Koga agar plate, ether-concentration, and Flotac for Schistosoma mansoni and soil-transmitted helminths. PLoS Negl. Trop. Dis. 4, e754.

Gonçalves, A.L.R., Machado, G.A., Gonçalves-Pires, M.R.F., Ferreira-Júnior, A., Silva, D.A.O., Costa-Cruz, J.M., 2007. Evaluation of strongyloidiasis in kennel dogs and keepers by parasitological and serological assays. Vet. Parasitol. 147, 132–139.

Gonzalez Akimori, D., Dalessandro, E.J., Nolan, T.J., Stieha, C.R., Lok, J.B., Stoltzfus, J.D.C., 2021. Transcriptional profiles in Strongyloides stercoralis males reveal deviations from the Caenorhabditis sex determination model. Sci. Rep. 11, 8254.

Gorgani-Firouzjaee, T., Kalantari, N., Javanian, M., Ghaffari, S., 2018. Strongyloides stercoralis: detection of parasite-derived DNA in serum samples obtained from immunosuppressed patients. Parasitol. Res. 117, 2927–2932.

Gottardi, M., Paula, F.M., Corral, M.A., Meisel, D.M.C., Costa, S.F., Abdala, E., Pierrotti, L.C., Yamashiro, J., Chieffi, P.P., Gryschek, R.C.B., 2015. Immunofluorescence assay for diagnosis of strongyloidiasis in immunocompromised patients. Infect. Dis. (London, England) 47, 550–554.

Graeff-Teixeira, C., Medeiros, E., Zanini, G.M., Brasil, C.A., Cardozo, B.L., Dalpiaz, M.G., Bisol, L.W., 1997. Inexpensive alternative material for the isolation of larvae with the Baermann method. Mem. Inst. Oswaldo Cruz 92, 399–400.

Grove, D.I., 1996. Human strongyloidiasis. Adv. Parasitol. 38, 251–309.

Grove, D.I., Northern, C., 1982. Infection and immunity in dogs infected with a human strain of Strongyloides stercoralis. Trans. R. Soc. Trop. Med. Hyg. 76, 833–838.

Hailegebriel, T., Petros, B., Endeshaw, T., 2017. Evaluation of parasitological methods for the detection of Strongyloides Stercoralis among individuals in selected health institutions in Addis Ababa, Ethiopia. Ethiop. J. Health Sci. 27, 515–522.

Hailu, T., Nibret, E., Amor, A., Munshea, A., 2021a. Strongyloides Stercoralis infection in Ethiopia: systematic review and meta-analysis on prevalence and diagnostic methods. Helminthologia 58, 17–27.

Hailu, T., Nibret, E., Amor, A., Munshea, A., Anegagrie, M., 2021b. Agar plate culture: an alternative sensitive routine laboratory detection method for Strongyloides stercoralis and hookworm parasites. Iran. J. Parasitol. 16, 72–80.

Hall, E., Lyriaki, M., Whitworth, F., Black, V., 2020. Severe strongyloidosis in dogs. Vet. Rec. 186, 354–355.

Harada, Y., Mori, O., 1955. A new method for culturing hookworm. Yonago Acta Med. 1, 177–179.

Hasegawa, H., Hayashida, S., Ikeda, Y., Sato, H., 2009. Hyper-variable regions in 18S rDNA of Strongyloides spp. as markers for species-specific diagnosis. Parasitol. Res. 104, 869–874.

Hasegawa, H., Sato, H., Fujita, S., Nguema, P.P., Nobusue, K., Miyagi, K., Kooriyama, T., Takenoshita, Y., Noda, S., Sato, A., Morimoto, A., Ikeda, Y., Nishida, T., 2010. Molecular identification of the causative agent of human strongyloidiasis acquired in Tanzania: dispersal and diversity of Strongyloides spp. and their hosts. Parasitol. Int. 59, 407–413.

Henriquez-Camacho, C., Gotuzzo, E., Echevarria, J., White Jr., A.C., Terashima, A., Samalvides, F., Pérez-Molina, J.A., Plana, M.N., 2016. Ivermectin versus albendazole or thiabendazole for Strongyloides stercoralis infection. Cochrane Database Syst. Rev. 2016, CD007745.

Hernández Chavarria, F., 2001. Strongyloides stercoralis: un parásito subestimado TT - Strongyloides stercoralis: an underestimated parasite. Parasitol. Día 25, 40–49.

Hernández-Chavarría, F., Avendaño, L., 2001. A simple modification of the Baermann method for diagnosis of strongyloidiasis. Mem. Inst. Oswaldo Cruz 96, 805–807.

Hoffman, W., Pons, J., Janer, J., 1934. Sedimentation concentration method in schistosomiasis mansoni. Puerto Rico J. Publ. Health 9, 283–298.

Hofmann, D., Sayasone, S., Sengngam, K., Chongvilay, B., Hattendorf, J., Keiser, J., 2021. Efficacy and safety of ascending doses of moxidectin against Strongyloides stercoralis infections in adults: a randomised, parallel-group, single-blinded, placebo-controlled, dose-ranging, phase 2a trial. Lancet Infect. Dis. 21, 1151–1160.

Holt, D.C., Shield, J., Harris, T.M., Mounsey, K.E., Aland, K., McCarthy, J.S., Currie, B.J., Kearns, T.M., 2017. Soil-transmitted helminths in children in a remote aboriginal Community in the Northern Territory: hookworm is rare but Strongyloides stercoralis and Trichuris trichiura persist. Trop. Med. Int. Dis. 2.

Huaman, M.C., Sato, Y., Aguilar, J.L., Terashima, A., Guerra, H., Gotuzzo, E., Kanbara, H., 2003. Gelatin particle indirect agglutination and enzyme-linked immunosorbent assay for diagnosis of strongyloidiasis using Strongyloides venezuelensis antigen. Trans. R. Soc. Trop. Med. Hyg. 97, 535–538.

Iamrod, K., Chaidee, A., Rucksaken, R., Kopolrat, K.Y., Worasith, C., Wongphutorn, P., Intuyod, K., Pinlaor, S., Sithithaworn, J., Sithithaworn, P., Hongsrichan, N., 2021. Development and efficacy of droplet digital PCR for detection of Strongyloides stercoralis in stool. Am. J. Trop. Med. Hyg.

Iatta, R., Buonfrate, D., Paradies, P., Cavalera, M.A., Capogna, A., Iarussi, F., Šlapeta, J., Giorli, G., Trerotoli, P., Bisoffi, Z., Otranto, D., 2019. Occurrence, diagnosis and follow-up of canine strongyloidiosis in naturally infected shelter dogs. Parasitology 146, 246–252.

Inês, E.D.J., Souza, J.N., Santos, R.C., Souza, E.S., Santos, F.L., Silva, M.L.S., Silva, M.P., Teixeira, M.C.A., Soares, N.M., 2011. Efficacy of parasitological methods for the diagnosis of Strongyloides stercoralis and hookworm in faecal specimens. Acta Trop. 120, 206–210.

Inês, E.D.J., Pacheco, F.T.F., Pinto, M.C., Mendes, P.S.D.A., Da Costa-Ribeiro, H., Jr., Soares, N. M. & Teixeira, M. C. A., 2016. Concordance between the zinc sulphate flotation and centrifugal sedimentation methods for the diagnosis of intestinal parasites. Biomedica: Revista del Instituto Nacional de Salud 36, 519–524.

Intapan, P.M., Maleewong, W., Wongsaroj, T., Singthong, S., Morakote, N., 2005. Comparison of the quantitative formalin ethyl acetate concentration technique and agar plate culture for diagnosis of human strongyloidiasis. J. Clin. Microbiol. 43, 1932–1933.

Jaleta, T.G., Zhou, S., Bemm, F.M., Schär, F., Khieu, V., Muth, S., Odermatt, P., Lok, J.B., Streit, A., 2017. Different but overlapping populations of Strongyloides stercoralis in dogs and humans-dogs as a possible source for zoonotic strongyloidiasis. PLoS Negl. Trop. Dis. 11, e0005752.

Jongwutiwes, S., Charoenkorn, M., Sitthichareonchai, P., Akaraborvorn, P., Putaporntip, C., 1999. Increased sensitivity of routine laboratory detection of Strongyloides stercoralis and hookworm by agar-plate culture. Trans. R. Soc. Trop. Med. Hyg. 93, 398–400.

Joseph, L., Gyorkos, T.W., Coupal, L., 1995. Bayesian estimation of disease prevalence and the parameters of diagnostic tests in the absence of a gold standard. Am. J. Epidemiol. 141, 263–272.

Júnior, A.F., Gonçalves-Pires, M.R.F., Silva, D.A.O., Gonçalves, A.L.R., Costa-Cruz, J.M., 2006. Parasitological and serological diagnosis of Strongyloides stercoralis in domesticated dogs from southeastern Brazil. Vet. Parasitol. 136, 137–145.

Kaewrat, W., Sengthong, C., Yingklang, M., Intuyod, K., Haonon, O., Onsurathum, S., Dangtakot, R., Saisud, P., Sangka, A., Anutrakulchai, S., Pinlaor, S., Cha'on, U., Pinlaor, P., 2020. Improved agar plate culture conditions for diagnosis of Strongyloides stercoralis. Acta Trop. 203, 105291.

Kalantari, N., Chehrazi, M., Ghaffari, S., Gorgani-Firouzjaee, T., 2020. Serological assays for the diagnosis of Strongyloides stercoralis infection: a systematic review and meta-analysis of diagnostic test accuracy. Trans. R. Soc. Trop. Med. Hyg. 114, 459–469.

Kato, K., Miura, M., 1954. Comparative examinations. JPN J. Parasitol. 3, 35.

Katz, N., Chaves, A., Pellegrino, J., 1972. A simple device for quantitative stool thick-smear technique in schistosomiasis mansoni. Rev. Inst. Med. Trop. Sao Paulo 14, 397–400.

Kearns, T.M., Currie, B.J., Cheng, A.C., McCarthy, J., Carapetis, J.R., Holt, D.C., Page, W., Shield, J., Gundjirryirr, R., Mulholland, E., Ward, L., Andrews, R.M., 2017. Strongyloides seroprevalence before and after an ivermectin mass drug administration in a remote Australian aboriginal community. PLoS Negl. Trop. Dis. 11, e0005607.

Khanna, V., Tilak, K., Prakash, P.Y., Mukhopadhyay, C., 2015. Modified agar plate culture method for culture of Strongyloides stercoralis. Trop. Parasitol. 5, 136–138.

Khieu, V., Schär, F., Marti, H., Sayasone, S., Duong, S., Muth, S., Odermatt, P., 2013. Diagnosis, treatment and risk factors of Strongyloides stercoralis in schoolchildren in Cambodia. PLoS Negl. Trop. Dis. 7, e2035.

Kightlinger, L., Kightlinger, M.B., 1990. Examination of faecal specimens by the formalin-detergent technique. Trans. R. Soc. Trop. Med. Hyg. 84, 417–418.

Knopp, S., Mgeni, A.F., Khamis, I.S., Steinmann, P., Stothard, J.R., Rollinson, D., Marti, H., Utzinger, J., 2008. Diagnosis of soil-transmitted helminths in the era of preventive chemotherapy: effect of multiple stool sampling and use of different diagnostic techniques. PLoS Negl. Trop. Dis. 2, e331.

Knopp, S., Salim, N., Schindler, T., Karagiannis Voules, D.A., Rothen, J., Lweno, O., Mohammed, A.S., Singo, R., Benninghoff, M., Nsojo, A.A., Genton, B., Daubenberger, C., 2014. Diagnostic accuracy of Kato-Katz, FLOTAC, Baermann, and PCR methods for the detection of light-intensity hookworm and *Strongyloides stercoralis* infections in Tanzania. Am. J. Trop. Med. Hyg. 90 (3), 535–545. https://doi.org/10.4269/ajtmh.13-0268. PMID: 24445211. PMCID: PMC3945701.

Ko, P.P., Suzuki, K., Canales-Ramos, M., Aung, M., Htike, W.W., Yoshida, A., Montes, M., Morishita, K., Gotuzzo, E., Maruyama, H., Nagayasu, E., 2020. Phylogenetic relationships of Strongyloides species in carnivore hosts. Parasitol. Int. 78, 102151.

Kobayashi, J., Hasegawa, H., Soares, E.C., Toma, H., Dacal, A.R., Brito, M.C., Yamanaka, A., Foli, A.A., Sato, Y., 1996. Studies on prevalence of Strongyloides infection in Holambra and Maceió, Brazil, by the agar plate faecal culture method. Rev. Inst. Med. Trop. Sao Paulo 38, 279–284.

Koga, K., Kasuya, S., Khamboonruang, C., Sukhavat, K., Ieda, M., Takatsuka, N., Kita, K., Ohtomo, H., 1991. A modified agar plate method for detection of Strongyloides stercoralis. Am. J. Trop. Med. Hyg. 45, 518–521.

Koga, K., Kasuya, S., Ohtomo, H., 1992. How effective is the agar plate method for Strongyloides stercoralis? J. Parasitol. 78, 155–156.

Koosha, S., Fesharaki, M., Rokni, M.B., 2004. Comparison of enzyme-linked immunosorbent assay and indirect immunofluorescence assay in the diagnosis of human strongyloidiasis. Indian J. Gastroenterol. 23, 214–216.

Kramme, S., Nissen, N., Soblik, H., Erttmann, K., Tannich, E., Fleischer, B., Panning, M., Brattig, N., 2011. Novel real-time PCR for the universal detection of Strongyloides species. J. Med. Microbiol. 60, 454–458.

Kristanti, H., Meyanti, F., Wijayanti, M.A., Mahendradhata, Y., Polman, K., Chappuis, F., Utzinger, J., Becker, S.L., Murhandarwati, E.E.H., 2018. Diagnostic comparison of Baermann funnel, Koga agar plate culture and polymerase chain reaction for detection of human Strongyloides stercoralis infection in Maluku, Indonesia. Parasitol. Res. 117, 3229–3235.

Krolewiecki, A.J., Ramanathan, R., Fink, V., McAuliffe, I., Cajal, S.P., Won, K., Juarez, M., Di Paolo, A., Tapia, L., Acosta, N., Lee, R., Lammie, P., Abraham, D., Nutman, T.B., 2010. Improved diagnosis of Strongyloides stercoralis using recombinant antigen-based serologies in a community-wide study in northern Argentina. Clin. Vaccine Immunol. 17, 1624–1630.

Kubofcik, J., Nutman, T.B., 2016. Next generation immunoassays provide one-step species-specificity for the diagnosis of filarial infections and strongyloides stercoralis in travelers and immigrants. Am. J. Trop. Med. Hyg. 95, 600.

Lau Chong, C., Samalvides Cuba, F., Terashima Iwashita, A., 2005. Evaluación de técnicas parasitológicas en el diagnóstico de estrongiloidiasis por Strongyloides stercoralis TT - efficacy of five methods for detection of Strongyloides stercoralis in human stool specimens. Rev. méd. hered 16, 11–18.

Le Pogam, A., Lopinto, J., Pecriaux, A., Fartoukh, M., Guitard, J., Voiriot, G., 2020. Strongyloides stercoralis disseminated infection in an HIV-infected adult. PLoS Negl. Trop. Dis. 14, e0008766.

Levenhagen, M.A., Fujimura, P.T., Santos, F.D.A.A., Vecchi, L., Alves-Balvedi, R.P., Madurro, A.G.B., Madurro, J.M., Costa-Cruz, J.M., Goulart, L.R., 2021. Innovative approaches to improve serodiagnosis of Strongyloides stercoralis infection. Braz. J. Infect. Dis. 25, 101545.

Lindo, J.F., Conway, D.J., Atkins, N.S., Bianco, A.E., Robinson, R.D., Bundy, D.A.P., 1993. Prospective evaluation of an ELISA and Western blot for the diagnosis of endemic strongyloides stercoralis infection - abstract. West Indian Med. J. 42, 50.

Little, S.E., Barrett, A.W., Beall, M.J., Bowman, D.D., Dangoudoubiyam, S., Elsemore, D.A., Liotta, J., Lucio-Forster, A., Mccrann, D.J., Snowden, K.F., Starkey, L.A., Tasse, S., 2019. Coproantigen detection augments diagnosis of common nematode infections in dogs. Top. Companion Anim. Med. 35, 42–46.
Llewellyn, S., Inpankaew, T., Nery, S.V., Gray, D.J., Verweij, J.J., Clements, A.C.A., Gomes, S.J., Traub, R., McCarthy, J.S., 2016. Application of a multiplex quantitative PCR to assess prevalence and intensity of intestinal parasite infections in a controlled clinical trial. PLoS Negl. Trop. Dis. 10, e0004380.
Lodh, N., Caro, R., Sofer, S., Scott, A., Krolewiecki, A., Shiff, C., 2016. Diagnosis of Strongyloides stercoralis: detection of parasite-derived DNA in urine. Acta Trop. 163, 9–13.
Lopez, M., Morales, M.L., Konana, M., Hoyer, P., Pineda-Reyes, R., White Jr., A.C., Garcia, H.H., Lescano, A.G., Gotuzzo, E., Cabada, M.M., 2016. Kato-Katz and Lumbreras rapid sedimentation test to evaluate helminth prevalence in the setting of a school-based deworming program. Pathog. Glob. Health 110, 130–134.
Loutfy, M.R., Wilson, M., Keystone, J.S., Kain, K.C., 2002. Serology and eosinophil count in the diagnosis and management of strongyloidiasis in a non-endemic area. Am. J. Trop. Med. Hyg. 66, 749–752.
Lumbreras, H., 1959. Aplicación de la Técnica de Baermann modificada en copa para el diagnóstico y control terapéutico. Rev. Med. Peru. 30, 21.
Lumbreras, H., 1963. Strongyloidosis: I. Evaluacion de la "tecnica de Baermann modificada en copa" en el estudiod e la strongyloidosis. Rev. Med. Peru. 22.
Lumbreras, H., Cantella, R., Burga, R., 1962. Acerca de un procedimiento de sedimentacion rapida para investigar huevos de Fasciola hepatica en las heces, su evaluacion y uso en el campo. Rev. Med. Peru. 31, 167–174.
Lutz, A., 1919. Schistosomum mansoni e a Schistosomatose segundo observações, feitas no Brazil. Mem. Inst. Oswaldo Cruz 11, 121–155.
Machado, E.R., Ueta, M.T., De Fátima Gonçalves-Pires, M.D.R., Alves De Oliveira, J.B., Faccioli, L.H., Costa-Cruz, J.M., 2003. Strongyloides venezuelensis alkaline extract for the diagnosis of human strongyloidiasis by enzyme-linked immunosorbent assay. Mem. Inst. Oswaldo Cruz 98, 849–851.
Machado, E.R., Faccioli, L.H., Costa-Cruz, J.M., Lourenço, E.V., Roque-Barreira, M.C., Gonçalves-Pires, M.D.R.D.F., Ueta, M.T., 2008. Strongyloides venezuelensis: the antigenic identity of eight strains for the immunodiagnosis of human strongyloidiasis. Exp. Parasitol. 119, 7–14.
Machicado, J.D., Marcos, L.A., Tello, R., Canales, M., Terashima, A., Gotuzzo, E., 2012. Diagnosis of soil-transmitted helminthiasis in an Amazonic community of Peru using multiple diagnostic techniques. Trans. R. Soc. Trop. Med. Hyg. 106, 333–339.
Maco Flores, V., Marcos Raymundo, L., Terashima, A., Samalvides Cuba, F., Miranda Sanchez, E., 2002. Fas2-ELISA y la técnica de sedimentación rápida modificada por lumbreras en el diagnostico de la infeccion por Fasciola hepatica. Rev. Med. Hered. 13, 49–57.
Marti, H., Koella, J.C., 1993. Multiple stool examinations for ova and parasites and rate of false-negative results. J. Clin. Microbiol. 31, 3044–3045.
Meurs, L., Polderman, A.M., Vinkeles Melchers, N.V.S., Brienen, E.A.T., Verweij, J.J., Groosjohan, B., Mendes, F., Mechendura, M., Hepp, D.H., Langenberg, M.C.C., Edelenbosch, R., Polman, K., Van Lieshout, L., 2017. Diagnosing polyparasitism in a high-prevalence setting in Beira, Mozambique: detection of intestinal parasites in fecal samples by microscopy and real-time PCR. PLoS Negl. Trop. Dis. 11, e0005310.
Miguel, C.B., Levenhagen, M.A., Costa-Cruz, J.M., Goulart, L.R., Alves, P.T., Ueira-Vieira, C., Brito, P.K.M.O., Gomes, A.O., Lazo-Chica, J.E., Oliveira, C.J.F., Rodrigues, W.F., 2020. scFv against HSP60 of Strongyloides sp. and its application in the evaluation of parasite frequency in the elderly. Dis. Markers 2020 (4086929).

Ming, D.K., Armstrong, M., Lowe, P., Chiodini, P.L., Doherty, J.F., Whitty, C.J.M., McGregor, A.C., 2019. Clinical and diagnostic features of 413 patients treated for imported strongyloidiasis at the Hospital for Tropical Diseases, London. Am. J. Trop. Med. Hyg. 101, 428–431.

Mircean, V., Györke, A., Cozma, V., 2012. Prevalence and risk factors of giardia duodenalis in dogs from Romania. Vet. Parasitol. 184, 325–329.

Mittal, S., Sagi, S.V., Hawari, R., 2009. Strongyloidiasis: endoscopic diagnosis. Clin. Gastroenterol. Hepatol. 7, e8.

Moghaddassani, H., Mirhendi, H., Hosseini, M., Rokni, M., Mowlavi, G., Kia, E., 2011. Molecular diagnosis of Strongyloides stercoralis infection by PCR detection of specific DNA in human stool samples. Iran J. Parasitol. 6 (2), 23–30. PMID: 22347284; PMCID: PMC3279873.

Mohammadi-Meskin, V., Hamedi, Y., Heydari-Hengami, M., Eftekhar, E., Sharifi-Sarasiabi, K., 2018. Is the Baermann, an applicable method for detection of Strongyloides stercoralis? HMJ 22 (2), 70–76.

Monteiro, M.F.M., Ramos, R.A.N., Calado, A.M.C., Lima, V.F.S., Ramos, I.C.D.N., Tenório, R.F.L., Faustino, M.A.D.G., Alves, L.C., 2016. Gastrointestinal parasites of cats in Brazil: frequency and zoonotic risk. Revista brasileira de parasitologia veterinaria = Brazilian journal of veterinary parasitology: Orgao Oficial do Colegio Brasileiro de Parasitologia Veterinaria 25, 254–257.

Montes, M., Sawhney, C., Barros, N., 2010. Strongyloides stercoralis: there but not seen. Curr. Opin. Infect. Dis. 23, 500–504.

Montresor, A., Mupfasoni, D., Mikhailov, A., Mwinzi, P., Lucianez, A., Jamsheed, M., Gasimov, E., Warusavithana, S., Yajima, A., Bisoffi, Z., Buonfrate, D., Steinmann, P., Utzinger, J., Levecke, B., Vlaminck, J., Cools, P., Vercruysse, J., Cringoli, G., Rinaldi, L., Blouin, B., Gyorkos, T.W., 2020. The global progress of soil-transmitted helminthiases control in 2020 and World Health Organization targets for 2030. PLoS Negl. Trop. Dis. 14, e0008505.

Moody, A., Rao, S. & Subirats, M. 2013. Evaluation of Parasep SF, *Ether and Ethyl Acetate Free Faecal Concentrators*, Apacaor: Berkshire, UK.

Moraers, G., 1948. Contribucao para o studo do Strongyloides stercoralis e da strongiloidosis no Brasil. Revista do Servicio Especial de Saude Publica 1, 507–624.

Mounsey, K., Kearns, T., Rampton, M., Llewellyn, S., King, M., Holt, D., Currie, B.J., Andrews, R., Nutman, T., McCarthy, J., 2014. Use of dried blood spots to define antibody response to the Strongyloides stercoralis recombinant antigen NIE. Acta Trop. 138, 78–82.

Nagayasu, E., Aung, M., Hortiwakul, T., Hino, A., Tanaka, T., Higashiarakawa, M., Olia, A., Taniguchi, T., Win, S.M.T., Ohashi, I., Odongo-Aginya, E.I., Aye, K.M., Mon, M., Win, K.K., Ota, K., Torisu, Y., Panthuwong, S., Kimura, E., Palacpac, N.M.Q., Kikuchi, T., Hirata, T., Torisu, S., Hisaeda, H., Horii, T., Fujita, J., Htike, W.W., Maruyama, H., 2017. A possible origin population of pathogenic intestinal nematodes, Strongyloides stercoralis, unveiled by molecular phylogeny. Sci. Rep. 7, 4844.

Nageswaran, C., Craig, P.S., Devaney, E., 1994. Coproantigen detection in rats experimentally infected with Strongyloides ratti. Parasitology 108 (Pt 3), 335–342.

Naidu, P., Yanow, S.K., Kowalewska-Grochowska, K.T., 2013. Eosinophilia: A poor predictor of Strongyloides infection in refugees. Can. J. Infect. Dis. Med. Microbiol. 24, 93–96.

Neimeister, R., Logan, A.L., Gerber, B., Egleton, J.H., Kleger, B., 1987. Hemo-De as substitute for ethyl acetate in formalin-ethyl acetate concentration technique. J. Clin. Microbiol. 25, 425–426.

Neva, F.A., Gam, A.A., Maxwell, C., Pelletier, L.L., 2001. Skin test antigens for immediate hypersensitivity prepared from infective larvae of Strongyloides stercoralis. Am. J. Trop. Med. Hyg. 65, 567–572.

Nielsen, P.B., Mojon, M., 1987. Improved diagnosis of strongyloides stercoralis by seven consecutive stool specimens. *Zentralblatt fur Bakteriologie, Mikrobiologie, und hygiene*. Series A, Medical microbiology, infectious diseases, virology, parasitology 263, 616–618.

Nilforoushan, M.R., Mirhendi, H., Rezaian, M., Meamar, A.R., Kia, E.B., 2007. A DNA-based identification of Strongyloides stercoralis isolates from Iran. Iran. J. Public Health 36, 16–20.

Noordin, R., Anuar, N.S., Juri, N.M., Wongphutorn, P., Ruantip, S., Kopolrat, K.Y., Worasith, C., Sithithaworn, J., Sithithaworn, P., 2021. Evaluation of a rapid IgG4 lateral flow dipstick test to detect Strongyloides stercoralis infection in Northeast Thailand. Am. J. Trop. Med. Hyg. 105, 688–691.

Norsyahida, A., Riazi, M., Sadjjadi, S.M., Muhammad Hafiznur, Y., Low, H.C., Zeehaida, M., Noordin, R., 2013. Laboratory detection of strongyloidiasis: IgG-, IgG4 - and IgE-ELISAs and cross-reactivity with lymphatic filariasis. Parasite Immunol. 35, 174–179.

Nutman, T.B., 2017. Human infection with Strongyloides stercoralis and other related Strongyloides species. Parasitology 144, 263–273.

Nyambura Njuguna, A., Kagira, J.M., Muturi Karanja, S., Ngotho, M., Mutharia, L., Wangari Maina, N., 2017. Prevalence of toxoplasma gondii and other gastrointestinal parasites in domestic cats from households in Thika region, Kenya. Biomed. Res. Int. 2017, 7615810.

O'Connell, E.M., Nutman, T.B., 2016. Molecular diagnostics for soil-transmitted helminths. Am. J. Trop. Med. Hyg. 95, 508–513.

Ottino, L., Buonfrate, D., Paradies, P., Bisoffi, Z., Antonelli, A., Rossolini, G.M., Gabrielli, S., Bartoloni, A., Zammarchi, L., 2020. Autochthonous human and canine Strongyloides stercoralis infection in Europe: report of a human case in an Italian teen and systematic review of the literature. Pathogens (Basel, Switzerland) 9.

Page, W.A., Dempsey, K., McCarthy, J.S., 2006. Utility of serological follow-up of chronic strongyloidiasis after anthelminthic chemotherapy. Trans. R. Soc. Trop. Med. Hyg. 100, 1056–1062.

Page, W., Judd, J.A., Bradbury, R.S., 2018. The unique life cycle of Strongyloides stercoralis and implications for public health action. *Trop med.* Infect. Dis. 3.

Pak, B.J., Vasquez-Camargo, F., Kalinichenko, E., Chiodini, P.L., Nutman, T.B., Tanowitz, H.B., McAuliffe, I., Wilkins, P., Smith, P.T., Ward, B.J., Libman, M.D., Ndao, M., 2014. Development of a rapid serological assay for the diagnosis of strongyloidiasis using a novel diffraction-based biosensor technology. PLoS Negl. Trop. Dis. 8, e3002.

Pampiglione, S., Ricciardi, M.L., 1972. Experimental infestation with human strain Strongyloides fulleborni in man. Lancet 1, 663–665.

Papaiakovou, M., Gasser, R.B., Littlewood, D.T.J., 2019. Quantitative PCR-based diagnosis of soil-transmitted helminth infections: Faecal or fickle? Trends Parasitol. 35, 491–500.

Papazahariadou, M., Founta, A., Papadopoulos, E., Chliounakis, S., Antoniadou-Sotiriadou, K., Theodorides, Y., 2007. Gastrointestinal parasites of shepherd and hunting dogs in the Serres prefecture, Northern Greece. Vet. Parasitol. 148, 170–173.

Paradies, P., Iarussi, F., Sasanelli, M., Capogna, A., Lia, R.P., Zucca, D., Greco, B., Cantacessi, C., Otranto, D., 2017. Occurrence of strongyloidiasis in privately owned and sheltered dogs: clinical presentation and treatment outcome. Parasit. Vectors 10, 345.

Paradies, P., Buonfrate, D., Iatta, R., Iarussi, F., Giorli, G., Palmieri, V.O., Sasanelli, M., Perandin, F., Šlapeta, J., Capogna, A., Otranto, D., Bisoffi, Z., 2019. Efficacy of ivermectin to control Strongyloides stercoralis infection in sheltered dogs. Acta Trop. 190, 204–209.

Pellegrino, J., Chaia, G., Memoria, J.M., 1961. Observations on the intradermal reaction to Strongyloides ratti antigen in strongyloidosis patients. Rev. Inst. Med. Trop. Sao Paulo 3, 181–185.
Perry, J.L., Matthews, J.S., Miller, G.R., 1990. Parasite detection efficiencies of five stool concentration systems. J. Clin. Microbiol. 28, 1094–1097.
Pilotte, N., Papaiakovou, M., Grant, J.R., Bierwert, L.A., Llewellyn, S., McCarthy, J.S., Williams, S.A., 2016. Improved PCR-based detection of soil transmitted helminth infections using a next-generation sequencing approach to assay design. PLoS Negl. Trop. Dis. 10, e0004578.
Polderman, A.M., Eberhard, M., Baeta, S., Gasser, R.B., Van Lieshout, L., Magnussen, P., Olsen, A., Spannbrucker, N., Ziem, J., Horton, J., 2010. The rise and fall of human oesophagostomiasis. Adv. Parasitol. 71, 93–155.
Porto, A.F., Oliveira Filho, J., Neva, F.A., Orge, G., Alcântara, L., Gam, A., Carvalho, E.M., 2001. Influence of human T-cell lymphocytotropic virus type 1 infection on serologic and skin tests for strongyloidiasis. Am. J. Trop. Med. Hyg. 65, 610–613.
Potters, I., Micalessi, I., Van Esbroeck, M., Gils, S., Theunissen, C., 2020. A rare case of imported Strongyloides fuelleborni infection in a Belgian student. Clin. Infect. Pract., 7–8.
Ramachandran, S., Gam, A.A., Neva, F.A., 1997. Molecular differences between several species of Strongyloides and comparison of selected isolates of S. stercoralis using a polymerase chain reaction-linked restriction fragment length polymorphism approach. Am. J. Trop. Med. Hyg. 56, 61–65.
Ramanathan, R., Burbelo, P.D., Groot, S., Iadarola, M.J., Neva, F.A., Nutman, T.B., 2008. A luciferase immunoprecipitation systems assay enhances the sensitivity and specificity of diagnosis of Strongyloides stercoralis infection. J Infect Dis 198, 444–451.
Ravi, V., Ramachandran, S., Thompson, R.W., Andersen, J.F., Neva, F.A., 2002. Characterization of a recombinant immunodiagnostic antigen (NIE) from Strongyloides stercoralis L3-stage larvae. Mol. Biochem. Parasitol. 125, 73–81.
Repetto, S.A., Alba Soto, C.D., Cazorla, S.I., Tayeldin, M.L., Cuello, S., Lasala, M.B., Tekiel, V.S., González Cappa, S.M., 2013. An improved DNA isolation technique for PCR detection of Strongyloides stercoralis in stool samples. Acta Trop. 126, 110–114.
Repetto, S.A., Ruybal, P., Solana, M.E., López, C., Berini, C.A., Alba Soto, C.D., Cappa, S.M.G., 2016. Comparison between PCR and larvae visualization methods for diagnosis of Strongyloides stercoralis out of endemic area: A proposed algorithm. Acta Trop. 157, 169–177.
Requena-Méndez, A., Chiodini, P., Bisoffi, Z., Buonfrate, D., Gotuzzo, E., Muñoz, J., 2013. The laboratory diagnosis and follow up of strongyloidiasis: a systematic review. PLoS Negl. Trop. Dis. 7, e2002.
Requena-Méndez, A., Buonfrate, D., Gomez-Junyent, J., Zammarchi, L., Bisoffi, Z., Muñoz, J., 2017. Evidence-based guidelines for screening and Management of Strongyloidiasis in non-endemic countries. Am. J. Trop. Med. Hyg. 97, 645–652.
Ridley, D.S., Hawgood, B.C., 1956. The value of formol-ether concentration of faecal cysts and ova. J. Clin. Pathol. 9, 74–76.
Riggio, F., Mannella, R., Ariti, G., Perrucci, S., 2013. Intestinal and lung parasites in owned dogs and cats from Central Italy. Vet. Parasitol. 193, 78–84.
Ritchie, L.S., 1948. An ether sedimentation technique for routine stool examinations. Bull U S Army Med. Dep. 8, 326.
Robertson, G.J., Koehler, A.V., Gasser, R.B., Watts, M., Norton, R., Bradbury, R.S., 2017. Application of PCR-based tools to explore Strongyloides infection in people in parts of Northern Australia. Trop. Med. Int. Dis. 2.
Rodrigues, R.M., De Oliveira, M.C., Sopelete, M.C., Silva, D.A.O., Campos, D.M.B., Taketomi, E.A., Costa-Cruz, J.M., 2007. IgG1, IgG4, and IgE antibody responses in human strongyloidiasis by ELISA using Strongyloides ratti saline extract as heterologous antigen. Parasitol. Res. 101, 1209–1214.

Ruantip, S., Eamudomkarn, C., Techasen, A., Wangboon, C., Sithithaworn, J., Bethony, J.M., Itoh, M., Sithithaworn, P., 2019. Accuracy of urine and serum assays for the diagnosis of strongyloidiasis by three enzyme-linked immunosorbent assay protocols. Am. J. Trop. Med. Hyg. 100, 127–129.

Rugai, E., Mattos, T., Brisola, A.P., 1954. Nova técnica para isolar larvas de mematóides das fezes - Modificação do Método de Baermann. Rev. Inst. Adolfo Lutz 14, 5–8.

Rutjes, A.W., Reitsma, J.B., Coomarasamy, A., Khan, K.S., Bossuyt, P.M., 2007. Evaluation of diagnostic tests when there is no gold standard. A review of methods. Health Technol. Assess. 11 (iii, ix-51).

Sadaow, L., Sanpool, O., Rodpai, R., Boonroumkaew, P., Maleewong, W., Intapan, P.M., 2020. Development of immunochromatographic device as a point-of-care tool for serodiagnosis of human strongyloidiasis cases. Eur. J. Clin. Microbiol. Infect. Dis. 39, 465–470.

Salazar, S.A., Gutierrez, C., Berk, S.L., 1995. Value of the agar plate method for the diagnosis of intestinal strongyloidiasis. Diagn. Microbiol. Infect. Dis. 23, 141–145.

Sandground, J., 1928. Some studies on susceptibility, resistance, and acquired immunity to infection with Strongyloides Stercoralis (Nematoda) in dogs and cats. Am. J. Hyg. 8, 507–538.

Sandosham, A., 1952. An investigation into the association of creeping eruption with Strongyloides infection contracted in the Far East. J. Helminthol. 26, 1–24.

Sanpool, O., Intapan, P.M., Rodpai, R., Laoraksawong, P., Sadaow, L., Tourtip, S., Piratae, S., Maleewong, W., Thanchomnang, T., 2019. Dogs are reservoir hosts for possible transmission of human strongyloidiasis in Thailand: molecular identification and genetic diversity of causative parasite species. J. Helminthol. 94, e110.

Santini, A., Lucchini, V., Fabbri, E., 2007. Ageing and environmental factors affect PCR success in wolf (canis lupus) excremental DNA sample. Mol. Ecol. Notes 7, 955–961.

Sato, Y., Otsuru, M., Takara, M., Shiroma, Y., 1986. Intradermal reactions in strongyloidiasis. Int. J. Parasitol. 16, 87–91.

Sato, Y., Kobayashi, J., Toma, H., Shiroma, Y., 1995. Efficacy of stool examination for detection of Strongyloides infection. Am. J. Trop. Med. Hyg. 53, 248–250.

Sauda, F., Malandrucco, L., Macrì, G., Scarpulla, M., De Liberato, C., Terracciano, G., Fichi, G., Berrilli, F., Perrucci, S., 2018. Leishmania infantum, Dirofilaria spp. and other endoparasite infections in kennel dogs in Central Italy. Parasite 25, 2.

Saugar, J.M., Merino, F.J., Martín-Rabadán, P., Fernández-Soto, P., Ortega, S., Gárate, T., Rodríguez, E., 2015. Application of real-time PCR for the detection of Strongyloides spp. in clinical samples in a reference center in Spain. Acta Trop. 142, 20–25.

Schär, F., Odermatt, P., Khieu, V., Panning, M., Duong, S., Muth, S., Marti, H., Kramme, S., 2013. Evaluation of real-time PCR for Strongyloides stercoralis and hookworm as diagnostic tool in asymptomatic schoolchildren in Cambodia. Acta Trop. 126, 89–92.

Schär, F., Inpankaew, T., Traub, R.J., Khieu, V., Dalsgaard, A., Chimnoi, W., Chhoun, C., Sok, D., Marti, H., Muth, S., Odermatt, P., 2014. The prevalence and diversity of intestinal parasitic infections in humans and domestic animals in a rural Cambodian village. Parasitol. Int. 63, 597–603.

Schär, F., Giardina, F., Khieu, V., Muth, S., Vounatsou, P., Marti, H., Odermatt, P., 2016. Occurrence of and risk factors for Strongyloides stercoralis infection in South-East Asia. Acta Trop. 159, 227–238. https://doi.org/10.1016/j.actatropica.2015.03.008. Epub 2015 Mar 17. PMID: 25795619.

Schnyder, M., Reichler, I.M., Eichenberger, R.M., Hofer-Inteeworn, N., Kümmerle-Fraune, C., Grimm, F., 2022. Strongyloides stercoralis in Swiss dogs - a retrospective study suggests an increasing occurrence of this potentially zoonotic parasite as a consequence of dog imports. Schweiz. Arch. Tierheilkd. 164, 89–104.

Sengthong, C., Yingklang, M., Intuyod, K., Hongsrichan, N., Pinlaor, S., 2020. An optimized agar plate culture improves diagnostic efficiency for Strongyloides stercoralis infection in an endemic community. Parasitol. Res. 119, 1409–1413.

Sharifdini, M., Mirhendi, H., Ashrafi, K., Hosseini, M., Mohebali, M., Khodadadi, H., Kia, E.B., 2015. Comparison of nested polymerase chain reaction and real-time polymerase chain reaction with parasitological methods for detection of Strongyloides stercoralis in human fecal samples. Am. J. Trop. Med. Hyg. 93, 1285–1291.

Siddiqui, A.A., Berk, S.L., 2001. Diagnosis of Strongyloides stercoralis infection. Clin. Infect. Dis. 33, 1040–1047.

Silva, L.P., Barcelos, I.S., Passos-Lima, A.B., Espindola, F.S., Campos, D.M., Costa-Cruz, J.M., 2003. Western blotting using Strongyloides ratti antigen for the detection of IgG antibodies as confirmatory test in human strongyloidiasis. Mem. Inst. Oswaldo Cruz 98, 687–691.

Sithithaworn, P., Srisawangwong, T., Tesana, S., Daenseekaew, W., Sithithaworn, J., Fujimaki, Y., Ando, K., 2003. Epidemiology of Strongyloides stercoralis in north-East Thailand: application of the agar plate culture technique compared with the enzyme-linked immunosorbent assay. Trans. R. Soc. Trop. Med. Hyg. 97, 398–402.

Sithithaworn, J., Sithithaworn, P., Janrungsopa, T., Suvatanadecha, K., Ando, K., Haswell-Elkins, M.R., 2005. Comparative assessment of the gelatin particle agglutination test and an enzyme-linked immunosorbent assay for diagnosis of strongyloidiasis. J. Clin. Microbiol. 43, 3278–3282.

Sitta, R.B., Malta, F.M., Pinho, J.R., Chieffi, P.P., Gryschek, R.C.B., Paula, F.M., 2014. Conventional PCR for molecular diagnosis of human strongyloidiasis. Parasitology 141, 716–721.

Speare, R., 1989. Identification of species of Strongyloides. In: D.I., G. (Ed.), Strongyloidiasis: A Major Roundworm Infection of Man. Taylor and Francis, Basingstoke.

Sprott, V., Selby, C.D., Ispahani, P., Toghill, P.J., 1987. Indigenous strongyloidiasis in Nottingham. Br. Med. J. (Clin. Res. Ed) 294, 741–742.

Stamey, J.D., Seaman, J.W., Young, D.M., 2005. Bayesian sample-size determination for inference on two binomial populations with no gold standard classifier. Stat. Med. 24, 2963–2976.

Steinmann, P., Zhou, X.-N., Du, Z.-W., Jiang, J.-Y., Wang, L.-B., Wang, X.-Z., Li, L.-H., Marti, H., Utzinger, J., 2007. Occurrence of Strongyloides stercoralis in Yunnan Province, China, and comparison of diagnostic methods. PLoS Negl. Trop. Dis. 1, e75.

Streit, A., 2008. Reproduction in Strongyloides (Nematoda): a life between sex and parthenogenesis. Parasitology 135, 285–294.

Štrkolcová, G., Goldová, M., Bocková, E., MojŽišová, J., 2017. The roundworm Strongyloides stercoralis in children, dogs, and soil inside and outside a segregated settlement in eastern Slovakia: frequent but hardly detectable parasite. Parasitol. Res. 116, 891–900.

Sudré, A.P., Siqueira, R.C., Barreto, M.G.M., Peralta, R.H.S., Macedo, H.W., Peralta, J.M., 2007. Identification of a 26-kDa protein fraction as an important antigen for application in the immunodiagnosis of strongyloidiasis. Parasitol. Res. 101, 1117–1123.

Sukhavat, K., Morakote, N., Chaiwong, P., Piangjai, S., 1994. Comparative efficacy of four methods for the detection of Strongyloides stercoralis in human stool specimens. Ann. Trop. Med. Parasitol. 88, 95–96.

Sultana, Y., Jeoffreys, N., Watts, M.R., Gilbert, G.L., Lee, R., 2013. Real-time polymerase chain reaction for detection of Strongyloides stercoralis in stool. Am. J. Trop. Med. Hyg. 88, 1048–1051.

Sykes, A.M., McCarthy, J.S., 2011. A coproantigen diagnostic test for Strongyloides infection. PLoS Negl. Trop. Dis. 5, e955.
Takano, Y., Minkami, K., Kodama, S., 2009. Cross infection of Strongyloides between humans and dogs in the Amami Islands, Japan. Trop. Med. Health 37, 149.
Tamarozzi, F., Longoni, S.S., Mazzi, C., Pettene, S., Montresor, A., Mahanty, S., Bisoffi, Z., Buonfrate, D., 2021. Diagnostic accuracy of a novel enzyme-linked immunoassay for the detection of IgG and IgG4 against Strongyloides stercoralis based on the recombinant antigens NIE/SsIR. Parasit. Vectors 14, 412.
Telemann, W., 1908. Eine Methode zur Erleich Terung der Auffindung von Parasiten-eiern In den Faeces. Dtsch. Med. Wochenschr. 34, 1510–1511.
Tello, R., Terashima, A., Marcos, L.A., Machicado, J., Canales, M., Gotuzzo, E., 2012. Highly effective and inexpensive parasitological technique for diagnosis of intestinal parasites in developing countries: spontaneous sedimentation technique in tube. Int. J. Infect. Dis. 16, e414–e416.
Thamsborg, S.M., Ketzis, J., Horii, Y., Matthews, J.B., 2017. Strongyloides spp. infections of veterinary importance. Parasitology 144, 274–284.
Tilli, M., Botta, A., Mantella, A., Nuti, B., Bartoloni, A., Boccalini, S., Zammarchi, L., 2021. Community-based seroprevalence survey of schistosomiasis and strongyloidiasis by means of dried blood spot testing on sub-Saharan migrants resettled in Italy. New Microbiol. 44, 62–65.
Uparanukraw, P., Phongsri, S., Morakote, N., 1999. Fluctuations of larval excretion in Strongyloides stercoralis infection. Am. J. Trop. Med. Hyg. 60, 967–973.
van Doorn, H.R., Koelewijn, R., Hofwegen, H., Gilis, H., Wetsteyn, J.C.F.M., Wismans, P.J., Sarfati, C., Vervoort, T., Van Gool, T., 2007. Use of enzyme-linked immunosorbent assay and dipstick assay for detection of Strongyloides stercoralis infection in humans. J. Clin. Microbiol. 45, 438–442.
Varatharajalu, R., Parandaman, V., Ndao, M., Andersen, J.F., Neva, F.A., 2011. Strongyloides stercoralis excretory/secretory protein strongylastacin specifically recognized by IgE antibodies in infected human sera. Microbiol. Immunol. 55, 115–122.
Vargas, P., Krolewiecki, A.J., Echazú, A., Juarez, M., Cajal, P., Gil, J.F., Caro, N., Nasser, J., Lammie, P., Cimino, R.O., 2017. Serologic monitoring of public health interventions against Strongyloides stercoralis. Am. J. Trop. Med. Hyg. 97, 166–172.
Verweij, J.J., Canales, M., Polman, K., Ziem, J., Brienen, E.A.T., Polderman, A.M., Van Lieshout, L., 2009. Molecular diagnosis of Strongyloides stercoralis in faecal samples using real-time PCR. Trans. R. Soc. Trop. Med. Hyg. 103, 342–346.
Watts, M.R., James, G., Sultana, Y., Ginn, A.N., Outhred, A.C., Kong, F., Verweij, J.J., Iredell, J.R., Chen, S.C.A., Lee, R., 2014. A loop-mediated isothermal amplification (LAMP) assay for Strongyloides stercoralis in stool that uses a visual detection method with SYTO-82 fluorescent dye. Am. J. Trop. Med. Hyg. 90, 306–311.
Watts, M.R., Kim, R., Ahuja, V., Robertson, G.J., Sultana, Y., Wehrhahn, M.C., Bradbury, R.S., Gilbert, G.L., Lee, R., 2019. Comparison of loop-mediated isothermal amplification and real-time PCR assays for detection of Strongyloides larvae in different specimen matrices. J. Clin. Microbiol. 57.
WHO, 2020. World Health Organization. Diagnostic Methods for the Control of Strongyloidiasis [Online]. https://www.who.int/publications/i/item/9789240016538.
Willcox, H.P., Coura, J.R., 1989. A new design of the Baermann, Moraes, Coutinho's technique for the isolation of nematode larva. Mem. Inst. Oswaldo Cruz 84, 563–565.
Willis, H., 1921. A simple levitation method for the detection of hookworm ova. Med. J. Aust. 2, 375–376.
Wright, I., Stafford, K., Coles, G., 2016. The prevalence of intestinal nematodes in cats and dogs from Lancashire, north-west England. J. Small Anim. Pract. 57 (8), 393–395. https://doi.org/10.1111/jsap.12478. Epub 2016 Apr 13. PMID: 27071856.

Wulcan, J.M., Dennis, M.M., Ketzis, J.K., Bevelock, T.J., Verocai, G.G., 2019. Strongyloides spp. in cats: a review of the literature and the first report of zoonotic Strongyloides stercoralis in colonic epithelial nodular hyperplasia in cats. Parasit. Vectors 12, 349.

Yang, M., Gebeheyu, E., Jung, S., Kwon, O., 2013. Treatment of naturally acquired strongyloides stercoralis infection in a dog with ivermectin. J. Anim. Plant Sci. 23, 337–339.

Young, K.H., Bullock, S.L., Melvin, D.M., Spruill, C.L., 1979. Ethyl acetate as a substitute for diethyl ether in the formalin-ether sedimentation technique. J. Clin. Microbiol. 10, 852–853.

Yunus, M.H., Arifin, N., Balachandra, D., Anuar, N.S., Noordin, R., 2019. Lateral flow dipstick test for serodiagnosis of strongyloidiasis. Am. J. Trop. Med. Hyg. 101, 432–435.

Zanzani, S.A., Di Cerbo, A.R., Gazzonis, A.L., Genchi, M., Rinaldi, L., Musella, V., Cringoli, G., Manfredi, M.T., 2014. Canine fecal contamination in a metropolitan area (Milan, North-Western Italy): prevalence of intestinal parasites and evaluation of health risks. Sci. World J. 2014, 132361.

Zendejas-Heredia, P.A., Crawley, A., Byrnes, H., Traub, R.J., Colella, V., 2021. Zoonotic soil-transmitted helminths in free-roaming dogs, Kiribati. Emerg. Infect. Dis. 27, 2163–2165.

Zhou, S., Harbecke, D., Streit, A., 2019. From the feces to the genome: a guideline for the isolation and preservation of Strongyloides stercoralis in the field for genetic and genomic analysis of individual worms. Parasit. Vectors 12, 496.

CHAPTER TWO

Advances in diagnosis of gastrointestinal nematodes in livestock and companion animals

Laura Rinaldi[a,*,†], J. Krücken[b,†], M. Martinez-Valladares[c,†], P. Pepe[a], M.P. Maurelli[a], C. de Queiroz[d,e], V. Castilla Gómez de Agüero[c], T. Wang[f], Giuseppe Cringoli[a], J. Charlier[f], J.S. Gilleard[d,†], and G. von Samson-Himmelstjerna[b,†]

[a]Department of Veterinary Medicine and Animal Production, University of Naples "Federico II", Naples, Italy
[b]Institute for Parasitology and Tropical Veterinary Medicine, Veterinary Centre for Resistance Research, Freie Universität Berlin, Berlin, Germany
[c]Instituto de Ganadería de Montaña (CSIC-Universidad de León), Departamento de Sanidad Animal, Facultad de Veterinaria, Universidad de León, León, Spain
[d]Faculty of Veterinary Medicine, 3331 Hospital Drive, Host-Parasite Interactions (HPI) Program University of Calgary, Calgary, Alberta, Canada
[e]Faculty of Veterinary Medicine, St Georges University, Grenada
[f]Kreavet, Kruibeke, Belgium
*Corresponding author: e-mail address: lrinaldi@unina.it

Contents

† These authors contributed equally to this work.

Advances in Parasitology, Volume 118
ISSN 0065-308X
https://doi.org/10.1016/bs.apar.2022.07.002

Abstract

Diagnosis of gastrointestinal nematodes in livestock and companion animals has been neglected for years and there has been an historical underinvestment in the development and improvement of diagnostic tools, undermining the undoubted utility of surveillance and control programmes. However, a new impetus by the scientific community and the quickening pace of technological innovations, are promoting a renaissance of interest in developing diagnostic capacity for nematode infections in veterinary parasitology. A cross-cutting priority for diagnostic tools is the development of pen-side tests and associated decision support tools that rapidly inform on the levels of infection and morbidity. This includes development of scalable, parasite detection using artificial intelligence for automated counting of parasitic elements and research towards establishing biomarkers using innovative molecular and proteomic methods. The aim of this review is to assess the state-of-the-art in the diagnosis of helminth infections in livestock and companion animals and presents the current advances of diagnostic methods for intestinal parasites harnessing (i) automated methods for copromicroscopy based on artificial intelligence, (ii) immunodiagnosis, and (iii) molecular- and proteome-based approaches. Regardless of the method used, multiple factors need to be considered before diagnostics test results can be interpreted in terms of control decisions. Guidelines on how to apply diagnostics and how to interpret test results in different animal species are increasingly requested and some were recently made available in veterinary parasitology for the different domestic species.

1. The needs of advanced diagnostic tools for gastrointestinal parasites of veterinary importance

Nematodes affecting the gastrointestinal tract are among the most common parasites in livestock and companion animals worldwide (Bellaw and Nielsen, 2020; Charlier et al., 2022; Inácio et al., 2021; Jürgenschellert et al., 2022).

Gastrointestinal nematode (GIN) infections are widespread in large and small ruminants, being attributed to different helminths such as

Haemonchus, *Ostertagia/Teladorsagia*, *Trichostrongylus*, *Cooperia*, *Nematodirus*, *Oesophagostomum*, *Chabertia* and *Bunostomum* (Kaplan, 2020; Matthews et al., 2016). GIN infections may influence animal health, welfare and productivity, in terms of reduced growth rate, meat, milk and wool quantity and quality, and reduced fertility (Charlier et al., 2020). The severity of infections is determined by several factors including the pathogenicity of the parasite species, single or mixed infections, the susceptibility and immunological status of the host, the infective dose and management conditions (e.g. type of pasture, temperature, rainfall, etc.) (Charlier et al., 2022).

Intestinal nematodes infecting horses include strongylines (large strongyles) and cyathostomins (small strongyles), as well as ascarids (i.e. *Parascaris univalens*), with high prevalence values worldwide (Ghafar et al., 2021; Scala et al., 2022). The large strongyles, occurring in the large intestine, consist of species undertaking somatic migration in the host (*Strongylus vulgaris*, *Strongylus edentatus* and *Strongylus equinus*) that cause severe pathological consequences and clinical signs due to the extensive migrations of developing larvae. Of these species, *S. vulgaris* is considered a major threat to equine health (Sallé et al., 2017). Cyathostomosis causes acute and persistent diarrhoea, colic, weight loss, fever and rarely mortality, mostly in animals up to 6 years of age (Corning, 2009).

Intestinal nematodes of pigs, e.g., the zoonotic species *Ascaris suum* and *Trichuris suis*, cause problems in reproduction and growth, with diarrhoea, poor feed conversion, and even death (Kouam et al., 2018). *Oesophagostomum dentatum* and *Oesophagostomum quadrispinulatum* (the nodular worms) may also be present but are generally considered less pathogenic (Nansen and Roepstorff, 1999).

The most common intestinal nematodes in dogs and cats are the zoonotic *Toxocara* spp., hookworms and *Trichuris* spp. (Traversa, 2011, 2012). The infection caused by these parasites may be sub-clinical, but it can become severe in puppies and in adults with high burdens (Maurelli et al., 2022). Also of zoonotic importance are infections with threadworm species such as *Strongyloides stercoralis* in dogs (Thamsborg et al., 2017).

The variety of parasitic infections caused by GI nematodes in farm and companion animals presents several challenges with regard to the development of innovative tools that are required for effective worm surveillance and control. Appropriate and accurate diagnosis has been a longstanding challenge for epidemiological screening and surveillance to provide information on control strategies and efficacy of anthelmintic treatments (Kotze et al., 2020; Papaiakovou et al., 2022).

By 2030, advanced diagnostic tools are expected to better guide the control of helminth infections in ruminants (Vercruysse et al., 2018), equines

(Nielsen et al., 2021), and companion animals (Nagamori et al., 2021), as well as in humans (Montresor et al., 2020; Stuyver and Levecke, 2021).

Despite conventional diagnostic techniques still having a predominant role in many veterinary parasitology diagnostic labs, the development and field implementation of advanced techniques for the diagnosis of GI nematode infections have developed rapidly in recent years. The last decade has brought important insight and updates in the parasitological diagnosis of intestinal helminth infections in animals and humans, paving the way to addressing the need for more sensitive diagnostic methods. The digital revolution has resulted in the development of new rapid, cheap and accurate point-of-care diagnostics with appropriate storage of the data, facilitating the rapid identification of infected animals or humans.

The review recently published by Papaiakovou et al. (2022), while assessing the strengths and limitations of existing methods applied to the diagnosis of GI helminth infections of humans and livestock, also provided insights into high-throughput sequencing approaches using barcoding and metagenomics-metabolomics.

In further untangling the portfolio of advanced diagnostic methods used in veterinary parasitology, the aim of this review is to assess the state-of-the-art in the diagnosis of nematode infections in livestock and companion animals and presents the current advances of diagnostic methods for intestinal parasites harnessing (i) automated methods for copromicroscopy based on artificial intelligence, (ii) immunodiagnosis, and (iii) molecular- and proteome-based approaches. Other diagnostic markers, i.e., pathophysiological and performance-based indicators, will not be considered in this review because they have been described elsewhere (e.g. Charlier et al., 2022).

2. Advances in copromicroscopy: Current situation and way forward

The simplest and most widely used method to detect gastrointestinal helminths in livestock and companion animals is the microscopic identification of parasite eggs (ova) in faecal samples (Cringoli et al., 2021; Nielsen et al., 2021).

After the foundation of copromicroscopy by C.J. Davaine in 1857, and the first description of faecal flotation by C.C. Bass in 1909 (Nielsen, 2021), several copromicroscopic techniques (and related tools and devices) have been developed. These include either qualitative methods, such as the direct simple flotation in a tube (Fülleborn, 1921) and the direct centrifugal flotation method (Lane, 1924), or quantitative techniques such as the Stoll dilution technique (Stoll, 1923, 1930), the widely used McMaster method (Gordon and Whitlock, 1939) and its improved modifications (MAFF, 1986), the Wisconsin flotation (Cox and Todd, 1962) and the recently developed FECPAK (www.fecpak.com), FLOTAC and Mini-FLOTAC techniques (Cringoli et al., 2010, 2017).

Several variants on the protocols of each of the above-described techniques have been proposed over the years and have been described in detail in manuals of diagnostic veterinary parasitology (e.g., Foreyt, 2001; Hendrix, 2006; MAFF, 1986; Thienpont et al., 1986; Zajac and Conboy, 2012).

Of these techniques, those used for the quantitative Faecal Egg Count (FEC) determination that assess the number of eggs per gram (EPG) of faeces are the most widely used, not only for epidemiological purposes and for selection of animals in need of treatments, but also to evaluate efficacy/resistance of anthelmintics through the Faecal Egg Count Reduction Test (FECRT) (Charlier et al., 2022).

In recent years, standard operating procedures (SOPs) and robust protocols of the FECRT have been successfully developed as a result of coordinated efforts by various international networks and funding organizations dedicated to animal health (Charlier et al., 2022). Standardized procedures have also been included by the World Association for the Advancement of Veterinary Parasitology (WAAVP) into the general guidelines for the evaluation of the efficacy of anthelmintics in food-producing and companion animals (Geurden et al., 2022) as well as into the specific guidelines for diagnosing anthelmintic resistance (AR) using the FECRT in ruminants, horses and swine (Kaplan et al., 2022).

For these reasons, the importance of copromicroscopic diagnosis has increased significantly over recent years, and several parameters have been thoroughly examined to evaluate the diagnostic performance of FEC techniques, e.g., diagnostic range, detection limit, sensitivity, specificity, accuracy, and precision (Cringoli et al., 2010, 2017; Nielsen, 2021) (Box 1). The choice of FEC method depends on the diagnostic/research purposes and has always represented a trade-off between the costs and ease of use on the one hand and the detection limit and other performance parameters on the other hand (reviewed by Levecke et al., 2012; Nielsen, 2021). Given the substantial variation in the performance of various traditional or improved FEC tests, no single technique is fit for all purposes and the choice of a technique depends on the intended objective and expected FEC within faecal samples (Ballweber et al., 2014; Ghafar et al., 2021).

BOX 1 Definition of the terms used in the chapter.

Terms	Definition	References
Detection limit	The multiplication (or conversion) factor of a given egg counting technique	Nielsen (2021)
Analytic sensitivity	The smallest amount of parasitic elements (e.g. eggs) in a sample that can be assessed accurately	Cringoli et al. (2010) and Nielsen (2021)
Clinical sensitivity (or diagnostic sensitivity)	The proportion of individuals that are correctly identified as infected as determined by a diagnostic method	Cools et al. (2019)
Specificity	The proportion of true negative samples that are detected as negative with the technique being evaluated	Nielsen (2021)
Accuracy	How well the observed values agree with the true values	Cringoli et al. (2010) and Nielsen (2021)
Precision	How well repeated observations agree with one another	Cringoli et al. (2010) and Nielsen (2021)
Technology Readiness Levels value (TRL)	A method for understanding the technical maturity of a technology during its acquisition phase. Designed initially by the National Aeronautics and Space Administration (NASA) as a method of assessing the maturity of a project and quantifying its relative risk of implementation was then applied to multiple industry sectors, including that of diagnostic devices	Beims et al. (2019) and Heder (2017)
SWOT (strengths, weaknesses, opportunities, and threats) analysis	A framework used to evaluate a company's competitive position and to develop strategic planning, assessing internal and external factors, as well as current and future potential	Teoli et al. (2021)
Artificial Intelligence (AI)	The ability of a machine to perform advanced functions, for instance, learning, decision-making, adaptation, control and perception	Borba et al. (2021)

BOX 1 Definition of the terms used in the chapter.—cont'd

Machine Learning (ML)	A sub-category of artificial intelligence (AI) that aims to teach computers how to learn and act without human intervention	Holzinger et al. (2020)
Deep Learning (DL)	A subset of machine learning (ML), where artificial neural networks (algorithms modelled to work like the human brain) learn from large amounts of data	Holzinger et al. (2020)
Target Product Profile (TPP)	The necessary characteristics of an innovative product to address an unmet parasitological need. TPPs could be used to better guide manufacturers in the development of 'fit for purpose' tests	Maurelli et al. (2020) and WHO (2021)

A wide range of factors can affect the FEC/FECRT results and might be related to underlying biological processes and the experimental design (pre-analytical phase), the FEC method (analytical phase), and/or the interpretation of results (post analytical phase) (Cain et al., 2021; Cringoli et al., 2010, 2017; Morgan et al., 2022; Nielsen, 2021; Slusarewicz et al., 2019) (Table 1).

There is consensus on the fact that improvements to traditional copromicroscopic methods might come from automation in data collection, analysis and reporting, which are known to be the most laborious and time-demanding steps (Stuyver and Levecke, 2021). As already underlined for medical parasitology, automation is not aiming to solve the methodological drawback of FEC techniques, but rather aiming to improve the accuracy of the readout and reducing the operational costs, both to processing samples and to reporting the results. The further development and marketability of automated systems will depend on the availability of image databases and the integration of engineering activities to overcome the shortcomings of the error-prone microscopic manual readout and reporting. Although image analysis for parasite eggs' recognition was demonstrated in the early 1990s (Mes et al., 2007; Sommer, 1996), automated FEC techniques have only

Table 1 Factors that may influence the pre-analytic and analytic phases of diagnosis.

Pre-analytic phase	Analytic phase
Modality to collect the sample (i.e. avoiding to collect the sample from the soil)	Choose of the technique based on: diagnostic range, analytic sensitivity, specificity, accuracy and precision
Quantity of sample collected	Homogenization of the sample to take the aliquot to analyse
Time before analysis	Choose of flotation solution (if required)
Modality of preservation of the sample	Experience of analyst
Choose of fixative to preserve the sample	Time to read the tool and count parasitic elements (PE)

been widely introduced within the past 5 years, thanks to the quickening pace of technological innovations in the field of diagnostics (Cringoli et al., 2021; Nielsen, 2021; Stuyver and Levecke, 2021). Thus, advanced systems for identification and counting of helminth eggs have been developed in order to reduce human errors and time of reading, so increasing diagnostic efficiency. These diagnostics are mostly based on semi-automated and automated systems (e.g. smartphone-based technologies, digital microscopes, etc.) combined with image analysis (e.g. FECPAK^{G2}, Lab-on Disk Platform, Kubic FLOTAC Microscope, etc.) for the detection of helminth eggs in animals and humans (Cringoli et al., 2021; Inácio et al., 2021).

Over the last decade, researchers have been working on digital image processing models and pattern techniques for the automatic recognition of parasitic elements (PE) in microscopic images. Initially, the studies were focused especially on the development of automated systems for the diagnosis of different parasites of public health relevance, e.g., soil-transmitted helminths, *Schistosoma* spp., and protozoa (Cools et al., 2019; Fernández-Rivas et al., 2021; Moser et al., 2018; Osaku et al., 2020; Vlaminck et al., 2019), with the ultimate potential to be expanded to all parasite species of veterinary importance.

Most of these techniques are based on artificial intelligence (AI), that is the ability of a machine to perform "intelligent" functions, for instance, learning, decision-making, adaptation, control and perception. To execute such functions, a classification process must be triggered so that scenarios can be identified, grouped and appropriately evaluated. Machine learning is a useful AI approach when this classification process depends on a huge data analysis. Machine learning has been used for epidemiological research, diagnosis and discriminating pathogens and to support taxonomic species discrimination in helminths (Borba et al., 2021). AI algorithms, including machine learning and deep learning, are used for the detection, segmentation, registration, processing, and classification of digitized parasitological images (e.g. helminth eggs).

Given the remarkable progress in these novel worm egg counting systems in recent years, there are reasons to expect that additional similar systems will be developed in the future, while these existing systems are likely to be refined, standardised and updated as well. Consequently, there will be an increasing need for validating and evaluating the qualitative and quantitative diagnostic performance parameters of these advanced systems and their modifications in the years to come (Nielsen et al., 2021).

The following sections provide a brief description of the advanced systems that are currently used for FEC and FECRT in ruminants, horses, pigs and companion animals. A SWOT analysis was performed, based on the scientific literature for each automated method, considering internal (**S**trength and **W**eaknesses) and external (**O**pportunities and **T**hreats) factors that could affect their commercialization (Table 2).

Furthermore, the Technology Readiness Levels (TRLs) value, a method for understanding the technical maturity of a product during its development phase, was calculated for some advanced techniques (Table 2 and Fig. 1). The TRL scale ranges from 1 to 9; 1 being the first step where the idea for a technology or service is conceived, to 9 where the final product or service is in the market where it receives feedback (Salazar and Russi-Vigoya, 2021).

2.1 Automated FEC techniques in ruminants

The use of reliable, low-cost, easy-to-perform FEC/FECRT methods to identify and quantify GIN eggs in faecal samples is of pivotal importance for ruminants, as well as for horses, where anthelmintic resistance is widespread and an alternative sustainable approach to helminth control is needed, which reduces the frequency of anthelmintic treatments, e.g., in the Targeted Selective Treatment (TST) strategy, in which treatment is based on individual animal health or production parameters (Charlier et al., 2022; Nielsen et al., 2021).

Unfortunately, traditional coprological methods, as mentioned above, could be a major limiting factor to the implementation and adoption of these approaches. For these reasons, a research priority should include the

Table 2 Semi-automated and automated systems for parasites detection (principle, the hosts from which samples were collected, the parasites detected, SWOT analysis, TRL and references).

				Internal factors		External factors			
Method	**Principle**	**Hosts**	**Parasites**	**Strenght**	**Weaknesses**	**Opportunity**	**Threats**	**TRL**	**References**
Mes	Systems of flotation to concentrate the eggs	Livestock	Gastrointestinal nematodes (GINs)	Not requires special equipment; fast in the analytic phase 24 samples in 40 min	It requires long time in pre-analytic phase	It represents the base for further implementations	Long preparation of the sample	1	Mes et al. (2001, 2007)
FECPAK[G2]	High-throughput technological system for *on-field* sample processing	Equids; Ruminants	GINs	Automated detection and count; remote parasite detection and data on line management; commercially available	Low accuracy; high costs	It may be used directly from farmers in field; new applications combined with nemabiome metabarcoding	Not easy to use; long preparation of samples to obtain the results	9	Mirams (2016), Rashid et al. (2018), Tyson et al. (2020), Boelow et al. (2022), and Reigate et al. (2022)
Automated robotic system	Based on an automated X-Y stage; trained convolution neural network analyses	Cattle; Dogs; Monkeys; Sheep	*Eimeria* spp.; *Isospora* spp.; Strongyles; *Toxocara* spp.; *Trichuris* spp.	Inexpensive (~US$350); portable; it does not require special sample preparation	The system can be used only with McMaster chamber	It may have a wide market	Only one validation for sheep and cattle	2	Li et al. (2019)

Telenostic system	Automated digital microscope with a $10\times$ lens using a machine learning software	Cattle	GINs	High level of agreement between the prototype and manual systems of FEC (i.e. McMaster and Mini-FLOTAC)	It requires long time to acquire and analyse the images ($\sim$42 min)	It may be used as semi or automated system, because it permits to store the images acquired and PE may be counted manually or by an algorithm	Validated only for cattle	8	Elghryani et al. (2020)
KFM	Automated digital microscope combine with Artificial Intelligence	Dogs; Ruminants	GINs; *Toxocara canis*; *Trichuris vulpis*	Perfect agreement with optical microscope counting $>$99% of recognizing PE; high sensitivity, specificity, accuracy and precision	Actually, not commercially available	It can be used directly in field; also fixed samples can be used; Possibility of remote control	A tutorial for the use may be required	5	Cringoli et al. (2021)
Parasight system	Based on a fluorescent egg staining and a smartphone to capture images	Goats; Horses; Sheep	Equine strongyles; *Parascaris equorum*; Trichostrongylid	2.5 min test time, less variable and more accurate than McMaster technique; commercially available	High cost; higher precision with low and medium levels, no with high level for sheep and goats	It may have a wide market especially for equine market	In sheep and goats has been alidated only for trichostrongylid	9	Slusarewicz et al. (2016, 2019, 2021), Scare et al. (2017), and Cain et al. (2020)

Continued

Table 2 Semi-automated and automated systems for parasites detection (principle, the hosts from which samples were collected, the parasites detected, SWOT analysis, TRL and references).—cont'd

				Internal factors		External factors			
Method	**Principle**	**Hosts**	**Parasites**	**Strenght**	**Weaknesses**	**Opportunity**	**Threats**	**TRL**	**References**
Lab-on-disk Platform	Based on a combined gravitational and centrifugal flotation and the use of a converging collection chamber to create a monolayer of eggs	Pigs	*Ascaris suum*	High-quality of images, permitting a good identification and count	High cost; potentially limited use in field, due to: (i) the need for a minicentrifuge; (ii) the need for electricity; (iii) relatively large size/ difficult to carry over distance	After an implementation it may have a wide market	Very difficult to use	1	Sukas et al. (2019)
Automated Diagnosis of Intestinal Parasites (DAPI)	Based on a motorised system to read slides, using a digital camera and a machine learning software	Dogs	*Ancylostoma* spp.; *Giardia* spp.; *Toxocara* spp.; *Trichuris* spp.	Automated detection of eggs through a machine learning software	High cost; not portable; not validated	It may have a wide market	More validations are required	1	Inácio et al. (2020)
VETSCAN IMAGYST	Composed by a digital slide scanner and a machine learning software	Cats; Dogs	Ancylostomidae; *Cystoisospora; Giardia*; Taeniidae; *Toxocara* spp.; *Trichuris* spp.	The system allows identification and count of eggs within 15 min; commercially available	High cost; not portable; specificity and sensitivity variable according to PE to detect	It is distributed by Zoetis, so it is easy to obtain	Validated only for dogs and cats	9	Nagamori et al. (2020, 2021)

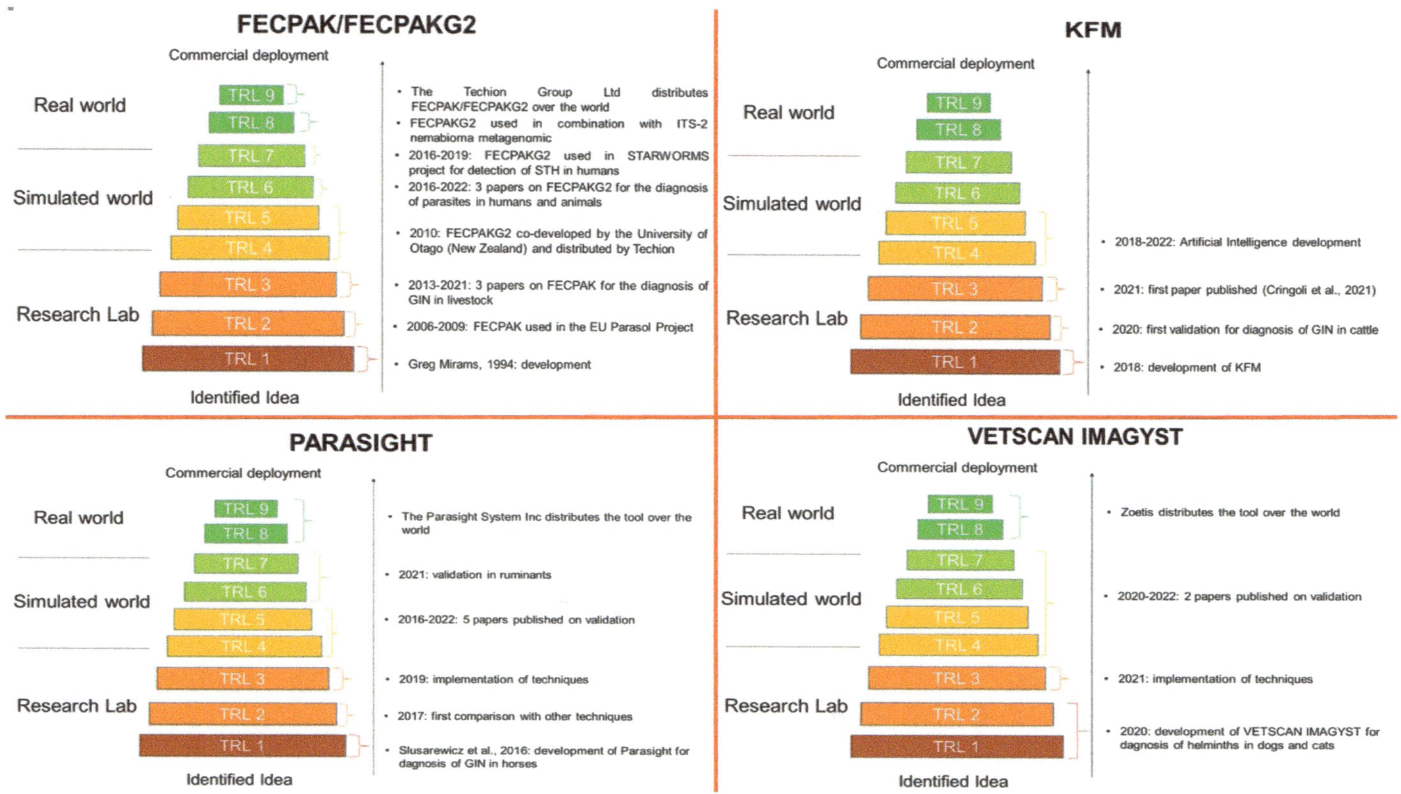

Fig. 1 Technology Readiness Levels (TRLs) value for each of the main automated FEC techniques used for the diagnosis of gastrointestinal nematodes in livestock and companion animals.

development of more standardised and user-friendly methods to obtain parasite egg counts for both pen-side and laboratory use (Rinaldi et al., 2019), including methods of automated sample processing and image analysis as indicated in the STAR-IDAZ (International Research Consortium on Animal Health; https://www.star-idaz.net) diagnostic road map for research on helminths and AR.

As reviewed by Inácio et al. (2021), initial studies on automated diagnostics involved the analysis of faecal samples from cattle (Sommer, 1996, 1998). In the first study, computer-assisted microscopy and multivariate statistics were used to establish and evaluate a procedure for identification of GIN eggs (*Ostertagia ostertagi*, *Cooperia oncophora*, *Haemonchus placei*, *Trichostrongylus axei*, and *Oesophagostomum radiatum*) in cattle, based on their morphological characteristics (i.e. shape and size). The percentage of correct classification for each species was: *O. ostertagi* 76.3%, *C. oncophora* 90.8%, *O. radiatum* 87.8%, *H. placei* 90.1%, and *T. axei* 83.8%, with an overall correct classification of 81.5% (Sommer, 1996). The procedure has been subsequently improved using the parameter of texture, which is the variation of the grey level in digital image processing, to identify GIN eggs. When texture was used together with the shape and size features, a higher percentage of eggs was correctly classified compared with the classification based on either texture, or shape and size. Therefore, all *O. radiatum* eggs were correctly classified as well as 88.3% of *O. ostertagi* and 91.2% of *C. oncophora*, with an average of 93.1% correctly classified eggs (Sommer, 1998).

A few years later, Mes et al. (2001, 2007) described a simple and robust method for digital recording and automated egg counting. They compared, initially, two techniques, Salt-Sugar Flotation (SSF) and Wisconsin Sugar Flotation (WSF) to identify the better method for isolating eggs, using egg-free faeces spiked with known numbers of GIN eggs, as well as faecal samples from naturally-infected cattle (Mes et al., 2001). The results showed that the SSF proved to be significantly better than the WSF, since it allows a larger number of samples to be processed and provides a high degree of precision (Mes et al., 2001). Once the eggs are isolated, they are concentrated in a very small area (1 mm^2), which allows digital recordings to be made, and the egg counting can be accomplished either manually or automatically. In the case of automated counts, a representative piece of the image is counted, the size of which depends on the number of eggs on an image. The algorithm used for the automated counts is based on parameters such as sphericity and size of the eggs, and it was shown to detect almost all of the eggs. As a consequence, the correlation between the observed number of GIN eggs and the expected number of eggs as determined by visual examination of eggs showed was very high (Mes et al., 2001, 2007). The limitation of this method is that if there are many thousands of eggs in a sample preparation, it is not possible to identify a representative section of the area due to aggregation of the eggs and, as a consequence, the amount of faeces needs to be reduced or the sample diluted. The GIN species of ruminants used to validate this method were *C. oncophora*, *Cooperia punctata*, *O. ostertagi*, *Trichostrongylus* spp., *Haemonchus* spp., *Oesophagostomum* spp. and *Bunostomum* spp. It is likely that the eggs of other helminths might be isolated using this protocol, adjusting, for example, the specific gravity (s.g.) of the flotation solutions (Mes et al., 2007).

FECPAK^{G2} is an image-based diagnostic platform, commercially available, for worm egg quantification in faecal samples, based on a flotation-dilution approach and on capturing digital images of samples without the use of a microscope. It has been developed for sheep and cattle, and other ruminants, as well as horses (Boelow et al., 2022; Rashid et al., 2018; Tyson et al., 2020) to replace the previously well-established FECPAK^{G1}, but it was also used in humans for automated diagnosis of soil transmitted helminths (Ayana et al., 2018; Cools et al., 2019; Moser et al., 2018). It was validated initially for counting GIN eggs in the faeces of alpacas using two flotation solutions (saturated sodium chloride and sucrose solution) and comparing performance with the McMaster technique (Mirams, 2016; Rashid et al., 2018). Results showed moderate to good agreement between the two techniques, with better agreement achieved when saturated sucrose was used as the flotation solution (Lin's concordance correlation coefficient$=$0.84), particularly when FECs were $<$1000 EPG. Recently, an improvement of the standard FECPAK^{G2} protocol has been evaluated, using sheep faecal samples, and shown to reduce the detection limit from 35 EPG to 5 EPG, thus making it more suitable for processing faecal samples with lower numbers of eggs (Reigate et al., 2022). In addition, an innovative application of the FECPAK^{G2} has been proposed by Francis and Šlapeta (2022). These authors have developed a new diagnostic approach based on the integration of FECPAK^{G2} with ITS-2 nemabiome metabarcoding, using a quick and simple protocol to harvest concentrated strongyle eggs through a repurposed pipette tip. The authors showed that nematode compositions, from FECPAK^{G2} egg nemabiome metabarcoding, are not different from traditional larval differentiation, and that FECPAK^{G2} eggs can be stored at room temperature in either lysis buffer or ethanol for up to 60 days, allowing for the transport of materials from remote locations in the absence of a cold chain (Francis and Šlapeta, 2022).

Li et al. (2019) developed an automated parasite diagnostic system consisting of a portable robotic microscope that can scan over the size of an entire McMaster chamber and capture high-resolution bright field images. The images are then automatically segmented and analysed using a trained convolution neural network (CNN). The system has been validated using faecal samples collected from different animal species (monkey, dog, sheep and cattle) and positive results were obtained for several parasites, including GI nematodes (e.g. strongyles, *Trichuris* spp., *Toxocara* spp.). The performance of the automated counting was then compared with a manual count by a trained operator for 28 samples containing strongyle eggs, and showed a high degree of concordance ($R^2=0.98$). Furthermore, the system was shown to be highly sensitive for mild infections. The overall accuracy of diagnosis using a 600 EPG diagnostic cut-off was up to 100% for nematode parasites (Li et al., 2019).

Telenostic is a novel, fully automated device for rapid quantitative field-diagnosis of cattle parasites (Elghryani et al., 2020). The Telenostic device is a prototype-automated digital microscope with a $10\times$ magnification. It is used in conjunction with a custom Telenostic cassette with a circular channel of approximately 2 mL capacity. Multiple images are acquired along the channel at the optimum focal point and these can be stored and made available for both manual and automated analysis of FECs. An algorithm for automated analysis has been developed to identify and count strongyle eggs. The Telenostic device has been compared with McMaster and Mini-FLOTAC for counting of GIN eggs in cattle faecal samples (Elghryani et al., 2020). Overall, consistent egg counts have been reported across the three devices and calculation methods, showing that the Telenostic device compared very favourably to the McMaster and Mini-FLOTAC techniques. Furthermore, both manual (laboratory technician) and automated analysis (image analysis algorithm) have been performed on the Telenostic device to calculate FEC. The results showed no significant differences between the automated and manual estimation of FEC with the Telenostic device, with high levels of agreement. However, little information is available regarding the further development and marketability of this technique subsequently.

The Kubic FLOTAC Microscope (KFM) is a compact, low-cost and portable digital microscope designed to analyse faecal specimens prepared with the Mini-FLOTAC/FLOTAC devices (and potentially suitable for other techniques) in both field and laboratory settings (Cringoli et al., 2021). The KFM combines the high sensitivity, accuracy and precision of the Mini-FLOTAC/FLOTAC techniques (Cringoli et al., 2010, 2017) with a reliable system to capture and analyse pictures. Moreover, the KFM can be remotely controlled by an external device, i.e., smartphone, tablet or PC. It is possible to transfer the captured pictures via internet to other laboratories, which could be very useful in creating a network or to support operators directly in the field. For KFM, an AI based predictive model has been developed to perform rapid, easy and precise automated recognition and counting of parasite elements/stages. The first validation of the KFM was performed on FEC of GIN in cattle. Faecal samples collected from cattle experimentally infected by GIN were analysed using the Mini-FLOTAC technique. Then, a comparison was performed between a traditional optical microscope (OM) and the KFM. The results showed substantial agreement (concordance correlation coefficient = 0.999) with low discrepancy between the GIN egg counts obtained (Cringoli et al., 2021).

The Parasight System is an automated method commercially available for horses (see below), which has recently been validated also in small ruminants (Slusarewicz et al., 2021). It is a smartphone-based automated parasite FEC technique that makes use of fluorescent staining and image analysis to identify and count parasite eggs in a sample without the use of a microscope (Slusarewicz et al., 2016). This system has been adapted for use with small ruminants, introducing a short centrifugation step in a flotation medium, an adjustment in pre-test sample filtering, and training of an image analysis-based egg counting algorithm to recognise and count strongylid eggs. The modified method has been compared with manual McMaster analysis using faecal samples from sheep and goats naturally infected with strongyle nematodes. The results showed comparable egg counts with the McMaster technique and no significant differences when comparing counts using faeces from either sheep or goats. Moreover, further comparisons, using sheep samples split into three groups based on strongyle egg counts (low, medium and high), showed good linear agreement ($R^2 = 0.958$) with egg counts determined with the McMaster method, but revealed significantly higher precision, as assessed by coefficients of variation, for the automated method for determining egg counts in the low and medium group (Slusarewicz et al., 2021).

2.2 Automated FEC techniques in horses

The emergence of AR, especially in equine cyathostomins, has led to the development of sustainable parasite control programmes based on systematic surveillance of egg shedding intensity (Andersen et al., 2013b). The surveillance-based methods consist in treating with an anthelmintic drug only those horses contributing the highest numbers of parasite eggs to pasture contamination (Nielsen et al., 2019). The principle of TST was meanwhile introduced in many horse farms and was often based on the treatment of horses with a FEC of strongyle eggs above a certain threshold (>200 EPG) (Nielsen et al., 2019). This emphasises the need for reliable and practical diagnostic tools to monitor egg shedding and anthelmintic efficacy via FECs (Tyson et al., 2020).

The Parasight system, as described above, is an automated parasite faecal egg counting device based on fluorescence labelling, smartphone image capture and computational image analysis (Slusarewicz et al., 2016). This technology makes use of fluorescent staining (chitin binding domain (CBD), from *Bacillus circulans* chitinase A1) and image analysis to count parasite eggs in a sample without the use of a microscope. Briefly, a device chemically processes a faecal sample and produces fluorescently stained parasite eggs via attachment of a fluorophore to chitin present in the egg surface. The stained eggs can then be photographed by a smartphone incorporated into an imaging unit. The smartphone then computationally analyses the image using an algorithm based on particle shape analysis to produce FECs. This system reliably identifies and differentiates strongyle from ascarid egg types based on the thresholds defined in the smartphone application (Slusarewicz et al., 2016). Furthermore, the time of processing has been reduced because the high-contrast images of stained ova can be identified at very low magnification, facilitating the imaging of a large amount of faecal material in a single photograph (approximately 10 times more than that contained in the two grids of a McMaster slide) (Slusarewicz et al., 2019). In addition, this method significantly reduces the technical variability compared with manual techniques (e.g. McMaster and Wisconsin) (Cain et al., 2020). The accuracy, precision, sensitivity and specificity of this new system has been compared with McMaster and Mini-FLOTAC methods, showing better precision than for the other two techniques ($P<0.0001$) and comparable accuracy with the McMaster method ($P=0.9411$). Furthermore, the system was significantly more sensitive (sensitivity, se = 94%) than the McMaster method (se = 55.5%), but it had significantly lower specificity (specificity, sp = 14%) than the other two methods (sp = 100% for both methods, Mini-FLOTAC and McMaster) (Scare et al., 2017). Thus, further refinements of the algorithm are needed to improve the specificity of this new FEC method.

The FECPAK^{G2} system, already optimised for sheep and cattle as well as for other ruminants (Rashid et al., 2018), was validated by Tyson et al. (2020) also for equids. The results showed that the accuracy of the G2 system, when compared with the G1, did not significantly change with rising FEC levels across a range of FECs of 100 EPG to over 3000 EPG. In addition, there was no significant difference between the egg count repeat samples using both methods. Recently, Boelow et al. (2022) compared the performance of a semi-quantitative sedimentation/flotation method with the quantitative methods Mini-FLOTAC and FECPAK^{G2} for detection of eggs of strongyles, *Parascaris* spp. and Anoplocephalidae. The results showed that the semi-quantitative sedimentation/flotation method turned out to be more sensitive than the quantitative methods Mini-FLOTAC and FECPAK^{G2}. Comparison of the results between the techniques showed almost perfect agreement ($\kappa \geq 0.94$) for the sedimentation/flotation method and strong agreement for Mini-FLOTAC ($\kappa \geq 0.83$) for strongyles and *Parascaris* spp. For FECPAK^{G2}, moderate and weak agreements were found for the detection of strongyle ($\kappa = 0.62$) and *Parascaris* ($\kappa = 0.51$) eggs, respectively. Despite the lower sensitivity, FECPAK^{G2} was able consistently to identify >90% of strongyle-positive samples above the arbitrary thresholds of EPGs at 50, 100 and 200 EPG based on all samples including negative ones. Thus, FECPAK^{G2} can be considered as an informative tool for treatment decisions against strongyle and ascarid nematodes in horses, particularly in cases where parasitological expertise is not available on-site (Boelow et al., 2022). Finally, the possibility to perform tests on-site makes it more convenient than other methods currently available, reducing the inaccuracies caused by the problematic storage of samples prior to testing (Tyson et al., 2020).

2.3 Automated FEC techniques in pigs

Pigs in modern and highly intensive pig production systems are usually infected with only a few worm species at low intensities thanks to a high level of hygiene (Nansen and Roepstorff, 1999). However, the new EU regulations for organic pig production require outdoor access to promote animal welfare, increasing the risk of infection with the common pig parasites, *A. suum* and *T. suis*, because their eggs can survive for many years in the soil (Lindgren et al., 2020).

As for ruminants and horses, worm control in the modern pig industry should be based on knowledge of the parasitological status and transmission capacity in the individual herd through routine surveys (e.g. coprological surveillance) to enable the design of parasite control strategies to mitigate the harmful effect of parasitism in pigs. To date, the lack of adequate coprological diagnostic tools for pigs has made the implementation of control programmes difficult. However, automated egg counting systems, based on computerised image analysis and deep learning algorithms, have been developed recently for parasitological diagnosis in pigs.

In 1999, Joachim et al. developed a method to differentiate morphologically fourth stage larvae (L4) of two species of porcine nodular worms, *O. dentatum* and *O. quadrispinulatum*, by computer-assisted analysis of digitised photomicrographs of L4 grown *in vitro* for various time periods and of L4 ex vivo. They demonstrated that morphometry could produce unbiased data which can be employed for the calculation of indices suitable for the differentiation of morphologically different specimens. The use of computer-assisted analysis of digitised photomicrographs of the two species facilitates the measurements of different parameters and subsequent data processing, offering the option for routine automated measurements (Joachim et al., 1999).

Recently, Das et al. (2019) described how two classifiers, the Multiclass Support Vector Machine (MC-SVM) and Artificial Neural Network (ANN), were used to identify *Ascaris* eggs in pig faecal samples. The accuracy rate for *Ascaris* egg identification using the MC-SVM and ANN classifiers was ~95% and 93%, respectively.

Finally, a lab-on-a-disk (LOD) technology for fast identification and counting of parasite eggs in pig faecal samples has been recently presented by Sukas et al. (2019). This technology includes a separation step to remove the solid particles, fat droplets and air bubbles commonly present in swine faecal samples. The separation is based on a combined gravitational and centrifugal flotation, with the eggs guided to a packed monolayer, thus enabling quantification and identification of subtypes of the eggs present in a single field of view. The prototype has been tested with faecal samples from pigs and humans infected with *A. suum* and other soil-transmitted helminths, respectively. For each experiment, the sample preparation procedure was performed in duplicate: one for testing in the LOD device and the other one for counting in a McMaster slide. Saturated sodium chloride (s.g. = 1.20) was used as the flotation solution for these experiments. The LOD device showed good performance compared with the McMaster method, showing egg recovery rates from 60% up to 100%. Finally, Sukas et al. (2019) have demonstrated that the quality of the images created by LOD was adequate for identification and quantification of egg types present in the faecal sample.

2.4 Automated FEC techniques in companion animals

Several methods are available to diagnose parasitic infections in companion animals. The sensitivity and limitations of each technique vary according to the parasite species, sample analysed, the technique itself and the level/experience of personnel (Sobotyk et al., 2021). For GI parasites, faecal flotation techniques are the most frequently used methods for detection of diagnostic parasite stages, mainly because of their low costs and because they are practical and direct, especially in clinical settings where a timely point-of-care diagnosis for intestinal parasites of dogs and cats is needed. Despite the benefits of routine laboratory microscopy examination, these tests are of low or moderate diagnostic sensitivity (Inácio et al., 2021). Computer-based algorithms to identify parasites in faecal examinations have been recently developed and introduced with the aim of improving the accuracy and reliability of coprological methods in dogs and cats.

The VETSCAN IMAGYST™ system is a commercial diagnostic platform that uses a combination of image recognition technology, algorithms and cloud-based AI to qualitatively detect parasite elements/stages. Initially, the system was tested to detect only four targeted parasites (*Ancylostoma*, *Toxocara*, *Trichuris vulpis* and family Taeniidae) in faeces of dogs and cats (Nagamori et al., 2020). An improvement of VETSCAN IMAGYST™ system is also able to detect intestinal protozoa (e.g. *Cystoisospora* oocysts and *Giardia* cysts) in faeces of naturally infected cats and dogs (Nagamori et al., 2021). The VETSCAN IMAGYST™ system consists of three main components: a sample preparation device, a digital microscope scanner, and a data analysis and reporting process. The VETSCAN IMAGYST™ faecal preparation device consists of two tubes: the sample tube with a sample scoop, which can hold approximately 1 g of faeces; and the collection tube containing two types of flotation solution, i.e. a zinc sulfate solution (s.g. = 1.18) for *Giardia* samples and a sugar-based solution (s.g. = 1.25) for the other parasites. The VETSCAN IMAGYST™ system can be utilised with either a centrifugal or passive faecal flotation process, although centrifugation significantly increases the sensitivity of faecal examination (Nagamori et al., 2020). The time-to-result of the full VETSCAN IMAGYST™ system including sample preparation, slide scan, and image analysis is around 14 and 10 min, respectively, for passive flotation and centrifugal flotation methods (Nagamori et al., 2020). Compared with conventional passive and centrifugal flotation methods, the diagnostic sensitivity and specificity of the VETSCAN IMAGYST™ ranged from 65.7–100% to 97.6–100%, respectively, across the targeted parasites. The VETSCAN IMAGYST™ has some limitations, such as the system does not examine the border or outside of a coverslip because of the predefined scan area (Nagamori et al., 2020, 2021).

Another system, developed in the Health Medicine and Computer Science areas at the University of Campinas (UNICAMP) in Brazil, is named "Automated Diagnosis of Intestinal Parasites" (acronym in Portuguese, DAPI) and consists of a parasitological protocol, computer and customised equipment containing a high-resolution digital camera, appropriate optical tube, and motorised stage (Inácio et al., 2020). The DAPI system was developed initially for the qualitative diagnosis of the 15 common species of human intestinal parasites in Brazil (Osaku et al., 2020; Suzuki et al., 2013) and then has been tested in a study involving four genera of canine intestinal parasites (*Toxocara* spp., *Ancylostoma* spp., *Trichuris* spp., and *Giardia* spp.) (Inácio et al., 2020).

The performance of a new parasitological protocol, named Prototic Coproparasitological (PC)-TEST DOG, has been compared against another technique, the Three Faecal (TF) test—GII/Dog and finally, the same slides were tested in the DAPI system to evaluate automated detection. The results obtained showed that the new technique (PC-TEST DOG) in combination with the DAPI system allowed a better visualization of the parasite structures, free of faecal residues, in dogs, especially regarding the egg and cyst identification of *Ancylostoma* spp. and *Giardia* spp. (Inácio et al., 2020, 2021). The PC-TEST DOG system needs further research to create a more robust database with images free of impurities and debris, so that the computer system can identify parasitic structure more accurately (Inácio et al., 2020).

More recently, an improvement of AI for the KFM, already validated for ruminants (Cringoli et al., 2021), has been achieved also for dogs. A dataset with 7802 objects, including samples of *T. vulpis* and *Toxocara canis* eggs recovered from faecal samples from dogs (confirmed by experts), has been used to train the software, proving that the AI system is able to recognise 99.0% of the eggs analysed (Maurelli et al., 2021). Therefore, the KFM might be a promising automated system for the rapid and accurate assessment of FEC to improve the diagnosis of parasitic infections in companion animals also.

As mentioned above for ruminants, Li et al. (2019) have developed an automated parasite diagnostic system. The image software has been trained also to recognise parasitic elements/stages (i.e. *Trichuris* spp., *Toxocara* spp., strongyles, *Isospora* spp. and *Eimeria* spp.) from other animal species, including dogs. The results have shown that this system can easily distinguish oocysts from eggs with high accuracy.

2.5 Future perspectives in automated FEC systems

Advances in technology and automated systems described above will likely change the parasitological diagnosis workflow, applying and developing AI models, so generating parasitological big data, and consequently moving forward the so-called teleparasitology. However, the diagnostic performance of these novel methods has mostly only been published as proof-of-concept results, without estimates of precision and accuracy (Cringoli et al., 2021; Elghryani et al., 2020; Inácio et al., 2020; Li et al., 2019; Lu et al., 2018; Nagamori et al., 2020; Sukas et al., 2019) and, as a consequence, further validation studies are needed using for example (i) spiked samples, (ii) composite reference standard methods, and (iii) Bayesian modelling (Nielsen, 2021). In addition, the further development of automated techniques may require the assessment of Target Product Profiles (Entrican et al., 2021) of the diagnostics that can make it to commercial application and increase their TRL.

3. Immunodiagnosis of gastrointestinal nematodes infecting farm and companion animals: From idea to market

Copromicroscopic diagnosis of GIN has some disadvantages and is sometimes accompanied by unreliable results, e.g., during the prepatent period, there is no egg shedding in faeces, and in addition, the egg count does not always correlate with parasite burden, and thus may not reflect the impact of the infection on animal health (Nielsen, 2021). In this context, and also taking into account that eggs of some GIN species cannot be differentiated microscopically, it is necessary to develop more sensitive and specific diagnostic methods. As described below, some methods have been developed in recent years that have allowed the detection of host antibodies or parasite antigens as markers of infection. Therefore, the measurement of antibodies resulting from an infection, or the detection of parasite antigens, could provide effective and sustainable markers as indicators for targeted selective treatments (TST), because they are easy to measure, ideally as a point-of-care method on the farm, and capable of assessing the health of the animals.

The immunological methods described to date for the detection of GIN infections in different animal species are discussed below. It is important to note that not all these methods are at the same stage of TRL. The TRL (Fig. 2) and SWOT analysis (Table 3) will be reported for the main immunological techniques.

3.1 Immunological methods for GIN in ruminants

As regards of *O. ostertagi*, enzyme-linked immunosorbent assays (ELISA) to measure antibody levels against a crude antigen of adult *O. ostertagi* have been used in epidemiological studies since the 1980s (Keus et al., 1981).

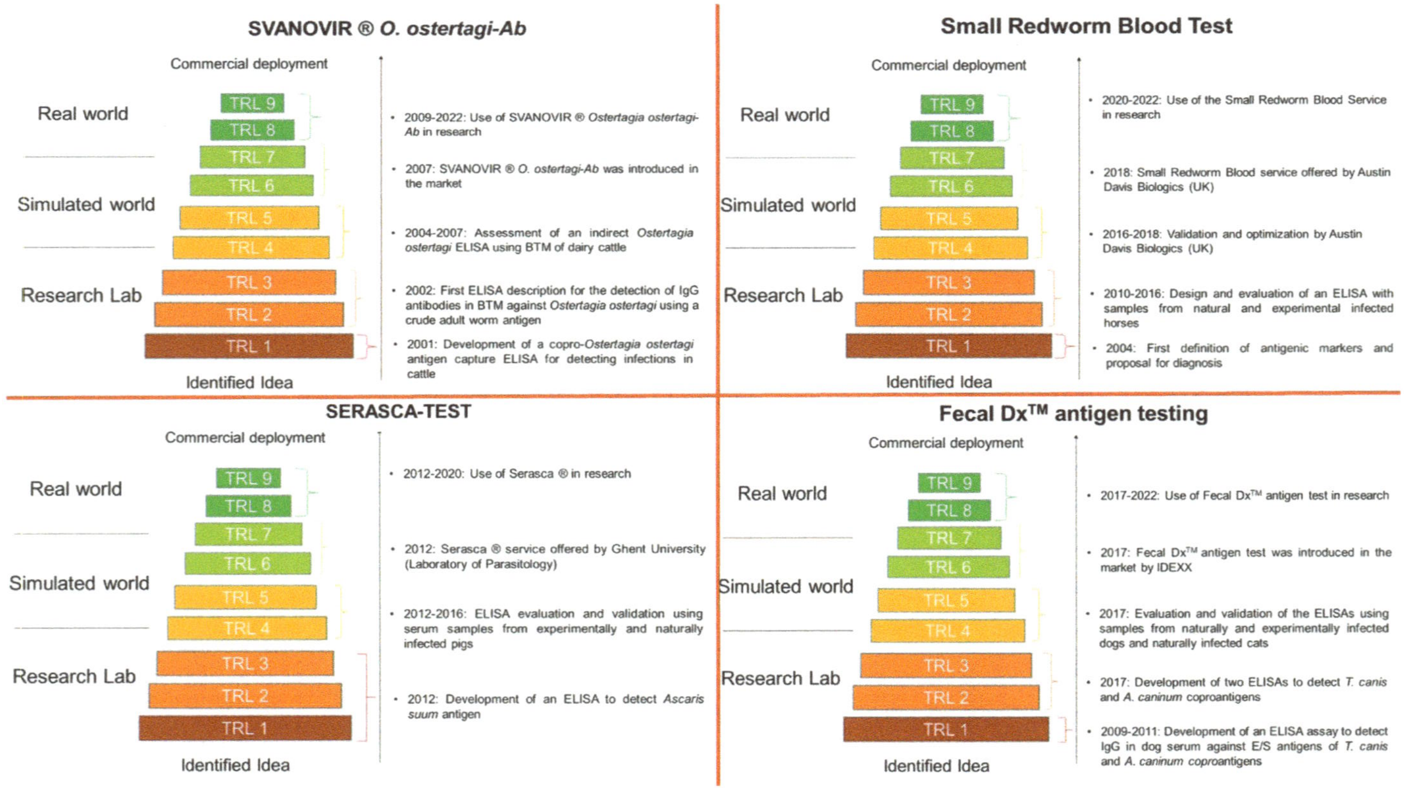

Fig. 2 Technology Readiness Levels (TRLs) value for each of the main immunological methods used for the diagnosis of gastrointestinal nematodes in livestock and companion animals.

Table 3 Commercialised immunological systems/services for parasites detection (principle, hosts, parasites detected, SWOT analysis and references)

				Internal factors		External factors		
Method	**Principle**	**Hosts**	**Parasites**	**Strenght**	**Weaknesses**	**Opportunity**	**Threats**	**References**
SVANOVIR *Ostertagia*	Detection of IgG antibodies inserum and milk	Cattle	Gastrointestinal nematodes (GINs)	Easy to perform	Need of a spectrophotometer	Can be used on serum or milk samples	A test quicker than this has been developed, but it is not yet commercialised	Charlier et al. (2007, 2009)
Small Redworm Blood service	A robotic system for detection of antigens in serum	Equids	Cyathostomins	No operator dependent	Geographically limited	If the service is implemented could be a wide market	Service only for UK submission	Walshe et al. (2021)
SERASCA	Detection of antigens in serum	Pigs	*A. suum*	Very sensitive and specific system	Geographically limited	It permits to detect a higher number of positive than copromicroscopic techniques	Service offered by Ghent University, Belgium mainly for vets in their country	Vlaminck et al. (2011, 2012)
Faecal Dx™ antigen testing	Detection of antigens in faecal samples	Cats; Dogs, Wolves	*A. caninum*; *T. canis*; *T. felis*; *T. vulpis*	Good sensitivity and specificity	Geographically limited	Available on market	Service for USA and Canada	Roldán and Espinoza (2009)

The assay quantifies the levels of immunoglobulins (Ig) G that react with crude protein prepared from adult-worm extracts of *O. ostertagi*. The assay was first used in the Netherlands to measure exposure to third stage larvae (L3) on pasture or the resuming development of arrested fourth stage larvae (L4) (Ploeger et al., 1995). Later, Sanchez et al. (2002) used and Charlier et al. (2005) measured the association between *O. ostertagi* antibodies in bulk tank milk (BTM) and parameters of milk yield and composition. These authors concluded that there is an important negative association between milk yield and *O. ostertagi* infection level estimated by this ELISA. The effect of anthelmintic treatment with eprinomectin on milk yield and BTM antibodies was also studied in herds naturally infected by different GIN species (Charlier et al., 2010). The deworming led to an increase in the kg/cow/day of milk during the 4 months after treatment but also a decrease in BTM antibodies; milk composition (percentage of fat and protein) was not affected by the treatment. Therefore, the authors reported that this *O. ostertagi* BTM ELISA is a useful assay to evaluate exposure to GIN and potential associated milk yield losses at the herd level (Charlier et al., 2007), so contributing to the targeted use of anthelmintics. The ELISA was further standardised and commercialised by Svanova (Sweden; now acquired by Indical Bioscience) allowing widespread availability and large-scale use. The commercial test, named SVANOVIR® *O. ostertagi*-Ab, was optimised to simplify the protocol; then, the within- and between-laboratory repeatability was assessed on different days and in four different laboratories (Charlier et al., 2009). The commercial ELISA has been used in several studies to determine the levels of exposure to *O. ostertagi* infection in different locations such as Mexico or Sweden (Frey et al., 2018; Höglund et al., 2010; Villa-Mancera et al., 2018), but also to predict the effect of anthelmintic treatment on individual milk yields (Vanderstichel et al., 2013).

A different immunodiagnostic test was designed to detect infection by *O. ostertagi* in beef cattle using non-invasive sampling, i.e., meat juice collected at abattoirs (Charlier et al., 2009). Although the assay highlighted a correlation between the presence of individual antibodies with a low carcass conformation score, cross reactions were described with other helminths (such as *Fasciola* spp. and *Dictyocaulus viviparus*), so that these associations may not show the effect of *O. ostertagi* exposure alone. More recently, Singh et al. (2019) developed a sensitive electrochemical immunoassay (e-ELISA) for the detection of *O. ostertagi* in serum samples. This approach is quicker than SVANOVIR® *O. ostertagi*-Ab kit, requires only 25 min, and has a better response, approximately fourfold higher. The next steps will be to advance in the development of immunosensors for e-ELISA, including validation with real samples to determine their reliability and reproducibility.

Regarding *C. oncophora*, not many immunodiagnostic assays appear in the literature. Karanikola et al. (2015) developed a multiplex fluorescence immunological assay (xMAP technology) for the simultaneous detection of antibodies against *C. oncophora*, *D. viviparus* and *F. hepatica* in cattle serum samples. The protein used for the detection of antibodies against *C. oncophora* was a 14.2kDa excretion-secretion protein (Poot et al., 1997) previously tested for herd health monitoring by an indirect ELISA (Githiori et al., 2000).

In sheep, local and peripheral antibody activity is related to GIN infection, with high levels of parasite-specific IgG1, IgE and IgA correlating with a low worm burden. Anti-parasite IgA activity in abomasal mucosa is associated with reduced worm growth and fecundity of the GIN species present in the abomasum such as *Teladorsagia circumcincta*, *Haemonchus contortus* and *Trichostrongylus colubriformis* (Hernández et al., 2016; Martínez-Valladares et al., 2005; Pernthaner et al., 2006). According to these studies, the correlation between gastric mucosal IgA and peripheral IgA in other samples such as blood, nasal secretions or saliva is positive and highly significant, ranging from 0.618 to 0.779. On the other hand, numerous studies have found an increase in IgA levels in animals or breeds identified as resistant with low FEC, although there is a high variability depending on the age of animals (reviewed by Aboshady et al., 2020). In sheep, specific IgA detection was not performed for diagnostic purposes, but as a marker in breeding programmes for animal selection since there is an intra- and interbreed variability in resistance to the infection (Hayward, 2013). However, quantification of GIN-specific IgA could be implemented as a diagnostic method after validating its usefulness within a specific breed. Measurement of specific antibodies in saliva or nasal secretions has the advantage of being a minimally invasive procedure relative to blood sampling. In these cases, detection of antibodies is frequently performed against L3, L4 or adult somatic antigen from different GIN species. However, Shaw et al. (2012, 2013) designed an ELISA assay to measure the IgA levels in saliva against a carbohydrate larval antigen (CarLA) present on the surface of the exsheathed L3 of all sheep GIN species tested to date. CARLA® saliva test is marketed by AgResearch (New Zealand) to measure the ability of sheep to respond to larval parasite challenge; animals with elevated levels of CARLA® antibodies have 20–30% lower FEC. Under low larval challenge during the season, CarLA-IgA was able to also reflect the exposure to GIN in cattle (Merlin et al., 2017). The value of measuring the level of specific IgA against GIN as a diagnostic method or as a marker within the TST strategy could be evaluated in the future.

In goats, there are not many studies describing the immune response and its association with worm burden as a preliminary step for the design of an immunodiagnostic method. For example, Basripuzi et al. (2018) did not find an association between increased anti-parasite IgA and FEC in the Boer goat breed, suggesting that the protective immune response in goats is ineffective or at least not IgA-associated. Similar results were previously shown by McBean et al. (2016) in Scottish Cashmere goats selected for low FEC; no consistent differences were found between specific IgA, IgE or IgG levels and FEC.

Regarding the detection of specific IgG against *T. circumcincta*, few studies reported its detection in milk samples, as a very easy to collect sample. Under experimental conditions, Cruz-Rojo et al. (2012) found that the association between specific IgG against *T. circumcincta* in individual milk samples and FEC varied depending on the time of lactation. In goats, Malama et al. (2014) described an ELISA for detecting antibodies against *T. circumcincta* in milk and serum samples with a sensitivity between 90% and 95% to detect the positive animals. However, when tested with respective sera from animals unambiguously infected with *F. hepatica* or *H. contortus*, cross reaction with antibodies against these parasites could not be excluded. More recently, Aliabadi et al. (2021) developed an indirect ELISA to detect infected sheep with worm burdens higher than 1000 adults by quantifying the specific IgG level against excretion-secretion *T. circumcincta* antigen in serum samples. Similar approaches were followed to measure the seroprevalence of *H. contortus* in sheep and goats using somatic and excretory secretory products from adult worms (Hassan et al., 2019; Kandil et al., 2017). However, the drawback of these assays was their poor specificity, showing cross reactions with other helminths such as *Fasciola* spp. or *Moniezia expansa*. In order to improve the specificity of these assays, Gadahi et al. (2016) identified the hepatocellular carcinoma-associated antigen 59 (HCA59), a excretory secretory product from larval stages of *H. contortus*, to measure the HCA59 IgG level in goat serum samples with a sensitivity and specificity of 87% and 100%, respectively (Naqvi et al., 2019). The same research group designed a different indirect ELISA to detect IgG antibodies against a tropomyosin of *H. contortus* in goat serum samples, with a diagnostic sensitivity of 90% and specificity of 100% (Naqvi et al., 2020). More recently, the immunodiagnostic efficacy of four glycoprotein fractions, i.e., Glucose, Galactose, N-acetyglucosamine, and Lactose, for the detection of anti-*H. contortus* IgG in sheep was evaluated (Toaleb and Abdel-Rahman, 2021). Indirect ELISA based on the Glucose fraction of *H. contortus* showed 100% sensitivity and 97% specificity in sheep serum samples (Toaleb and Abdel-Rahman, 2021). The value of these ELISAs must be further evaluated under field conditions.

3.2 Immunological methods for intestinal nematodes in horses

S. vulgaris is considered the most pathogenic parasite infecting horses. Detection of infection is complicated by the long prepatent period of six months during which the larvae migrate through the cranial mesenteric artery and its main branches, which can lead to verminous endarteritis, eventual thromboembolism and colic (Reinemeyer and Nielsen, 2009). Andersen et al. (2013a) described an ELISA using a polypeptide of the excretory-secretory fraction of the migrating larvae, named SvSXP, for detecting the level of antigen specific IgG(T) antibodies in serum with a sensitivity and specificity of 73.3% and 81.0%, respectively. Nielsen et al. (2014) confirmed a significant association between these ELISA values and larval *S. vulgaris* burdens ($P < 0.0001$). Later, Nielsen et al. (2015) showed that ELISA values were indicative of current *S. vulgaris* infection or previous exposure in the last 5 months. The demonstration of this assay in an operational environment was conducted in rural regions of Kentucky to study the prevalence of the infection, and in a prospective case-control study including more than 600 equine clinic patients (Gehlen et al., 2020; Scare et al., 2018). Recent studies from Germany also reported high frequencies of exposure to *S. vulgaris* using this ELISA (Jürgenschellert et al., 2022). Furthermore, authors suggested its value in diagnosis and management of horses with colic (Nielsen et al., 2016). On the other hand, some attempts have been made to detect *S. vulgaris* infection in non-invasive samples such as faeces by measuring total IgA (Tombak et al., 2020). These authors found that strongyle nematode FEC correlated significantly with total IgA in donkeys but only when body condition was uniformly good.

As for cyathostomins, encysted larvae embedded in the mucosa/submucosa of the colon and caecum can emerge synchronously in the lumen of the intestine and cause larval cyathostominosis. This syndrome, although uncommon, can be fatal in up to 50% of cases, however, there is no practical diagnostic method available for the *in vivo* detection of encysted larvae (Matthews, 2008). For this purpose, Dowdall et al. (2004) identified two native antigen complexes that showed utility as diagnostic markers for the indirect estimation of cyathostomin encysted larval burden, one of them being a protein named cyathostomin gut-associated larval antigen-1 (Cy-GALA-1), and the target of serum IgG(T) antibodies in experimentally- and naturally-infected horses (McWilliam et al., 2010; Mitchell et al., 2016). More recently, Tzelos et al. (2020), tested individual Cy-CID and Cy-GALA proteins and three multi-antigen cocktails comprising variations of the antigens from different cyathostomin species by measuring the specific IgG(G) levels in serum. A combination of proteins from the most common cyathostomin species, *Cyathostomum catinatum*, *Cylicocyclus nassatus* and *Cylicostephanus longibursatus*, had the best predictive value for infection. This assay, developed by Tzelos et al. (2020), was suggested for use in northern temperate regions in autumn/early winter to inform the need for larvicidal treatment at the end of the grazing season in animals at moderate to high risk. In parallel, the test was validated and optimised by the company Austin Davis Biologics Ltd. (UK) in a robotic system. This diagnostic service was launched in September 2019 as "Small Redworm Blood Test" (https://www.austindavis.co.uk/small-redworm-blood-test). In addition, guidelines for interpreting ELISA results have been implemented, taking into account previous coprological analyses performed at different grazing times. Diagnosis of infection in an outbreak in November 2018 in Ireland was possible following analysis of serological samples using this cyathostomin-specific ELISA (Walshe et al., 2021). The different phases through which this service has passed until its marketing are shown in Fig. 2.

Parascaris univalens is a nematode found ubiquitously in young equids. Although infection can be diagnosed by microscopic detection of eggs 10–15 weeks after infection, pathology and respiratory signs may appear during the migratory phase (Clayton, 1986). Therefore, correct diagnosis is essential during the prepatent period. In this respect, some antigens from the excretion-secretion products of third larval stage were identified in order to develop an immunodiagnostic test for prepatent diagnostic testing (Burk et al., 2014). These antigens were recognised in sera from foals naturally infected with *P. univalens* by measuring specific IgG(T) antibodies; however, the passive transfer of colostral antibodies from mares to foals could limit the value of the test (Burk et al., 2016).

3.3 Immunological methods for intestinal nematodes in pigs

Several indirect ELISA assays were developed in the past using protein extracts or excretory–secretory products of *A. suum* larvae or adult worms

(Bøgh et al., 1994; Frontera et al., 2003; Roepstorff, 1998). Vlaminck et al. (2012) later developed a serological test based on the immunological detection of *A. suum* haemoglobin antigen (As-Hb) (Vlaminck et al., 2011). The ELISA was validated with serum samples from experimentally and naturally infected pigs, showing a sensitivity and specificity of 99.5% and 100%, respectively; cross-reactions with *T. suis*-positive serum samples was limited. This ELISA has been used to measure the level of exposure to the infection on fattening farms in Germany, Belgium, Spain or China, as well as to determine the negative impact of the infection on production parameters (Lassen et al., 2019; Martínez-Pérez et al., 2017; Vlaminck et al., 2015; Zheng et al., 2020). In these studies, herds with higher antibody levels showed lower average daily weight gain, higher percentage of livers rejected due to milk spots caused by migrating larvae, and more severe clinical respiratory symptoms. Other applications of this assay have been the measurement of exposure of piglets to *A. suum* during the nursery phase (Vandekerckhove et al., 2017), or antibody monitoring after a 6-weekly treatment programme with fenbendazole in fattening pigs (Vandekerckhove et al., 2019). This As-Hb-based ELISA is currently marketed in Europe by Ghent University under the name SERASCA® for the diagnosis of *Ascaris* infection pressure in fattening pigs (http://www.serasca.com/en/Home). Recently, Joachim et al. (2021) evaluated the seroprevalence of *A. suum* infection in pigs from conventional indoor breeding systems in Austria by SERASCA®.

The same research group who developed SERASCA® also designed a different serological test based on recognition of the water-soluble protein extract of lung stage L3s of *A. suum* (As-Lung-L3 ELISA) (Vandekerckhove et al., 2017). This test showed a sensitivity of 90% and a specificity of 99% in serum from piglets infected with a minimum dose of 20 *A. suum* eggs/day and above over 7 consecutive weeks; however, when piglets were infected with 10 eggs/day, the sensitivity of the test decreased substantially. In an attempt to identify new antigens for novel serodiagnostic methods, Vlaminck et al. (2016) identified one major immunodominant antigen in the extracts and excretion-secretion material of infective *Ascaris* L3, a glycolipid, named As12. Experimentally infected pigs, and humans naturally infected with *Ascaris lumbricoides*, developed antibodies against the antigen As12. Based on SERASCA®, the ELISA kit Monoscreen™ AbELISA *Ascaris suum* (Bio-X Diagnostics, Belgium) is commercially available for the detection of serum antibodies directed against larvae and adult worms.

In addition, some in-house ELISAs have been developed to detect antibodies against *A. suum* infections in tissue fluids after a muscle freeze/thaw process. Thakur et al. (2013) used excretion-secretion products from

A. suum adult worms as well as from *T. suis* to determine the seroprevalence of both infections in indoor conventionally raised and outdoor swine. Helminth excretion-secretion products were used to quantify the specific antibody response (IgG1 and IgG2) in serum samples from pigs experimentally infected by *T. suis* and *O. dentatum* (Andreasen et al., 2015). Kringel et al. (2015) reported a significant correlation between *T. suis* FEC and specific IgG2 levels using excretion-secretion antigen at days 7 and 14 post-infection. However, the value of this assay as a diagnostic tool should be examined under field conditions.

3.4 Immunological methods for intestinal nematodes in dogs and cats

A serodiagnostic assay to detect specific-IgG against *T. canis* was developed by Regis et al. (2011) using larval excretion-secretion products to study the risk factors for the infection in dogs from Brazil. According to previous research (Roldán and Espinoza, 2009), the excretory-secretory products from *T. canis* cross react with antibodies against *A. caninum*. Therefore, in the study conducted by Regis et al. (2011), the dog sera were incubated with *A. caninum* antigen before performing the ELISA to adsorb cross-reactive IgG antibodies. Despite this, this assay showed low sensitivity (79%) and specificity (40%) when specific-IgG levels were compared with microscopy and PCR (Jarad et al., 2019).

3.5 Future perspectives in coproantigen detection and proteomics

Diagnosis of an infection can also be done by the detection of parasite antigens in faeces, i.e., by coproantigen ELISA. Coproantigen detection methods have the advantage that they do not rely on an exponential amplification process such as PCR and they are therefore less likely to have high frequencies of false positives due to contamination of samples or reactions. They can often be performed using ELISA formats established in almost all diagnostic laboratories and can also be applied pen-side or as point-of-care tests using, e.g., lateral flow formats. For human GINs, detection of hookworms (Bungiro and Cappello, 2005), *A. lumbricoides* (Lagatie et al., 2020) and *S. stercoralis* (El-Badry, 2009; Sykes and McCarthy, 2011) has been described. Elsemore et al. (2017) developed two different assays for dogs, one for detecting *T. canis* coproantigen and the other for *A. caninum*. For that, polyclonal and monoclonal antibodies were produced against recombinantly expressed *A. caninum* Asp-5 protein (Zhan et al., 2003) and a *T. canis* protease inhibitor homologue (Peanasky et al., 1984). ELISAs were validated with samples from dogs with experimental and natural infections. In the experimental infection, the *T. canis* coproantigen values dropped to negative status after an anthelmintic treatment; however, *A. caninum* coproantigen levels became positive at day 16 after treatment, with no eggs in faeces. According to the authors, this rise in antigen level could indicate the presence of worms sequestered in tissue at the time of treatment, which could have repopulated the intestinal lumen later (Elsemore et al., 2017). Furthermore, both ELISAs were also validated with samples from naturally infected cats, showing that it is possible to detect the feline counterparts, *Ancylostoma tubaeforme* and *Toxocara cati*. The test for ascarids also detects the racoon parasite *Baylisascaris procyonis* (Sapp et al., 2020).

Elsemore et al. (2014) designed an ELISA for coproantigen detection of infection using monoclonal antibodies against a recombinant whipworm (*Trichuris vulpis*) porin protein. Coproantigens were detected in faeces in experimentally infected dogs from day 23 post-infection onwards and no cross reactions were observed with positive samples for *T. canis* or *A. caninum*. The sensitivity and specificity of the three ELISAs for coproantigen detection was reported by Adolph et al. (2017) after comparing the coproantigen levels with microscopic observations after centrifugal flotation and necropsy. The values obtained for each coproantigen ELISA were 66.7% sensitivity and 100% specificity in the *T. canis* assay; 97.7% and 83.3% in the assay for *A. caninum* detection and 72.2% sensitivity and 98.2% specificity in the *T. vulpis* assay. For canine samples, only moderate agreement was observed between coproantigen ELISAs and sensitive flotation followed by microscopic diagnosis by an experienced examiner (Little et al., 2019). Reasons for a lack of agreement between the two methods might be collection of a sample during the pre-patent period before egg shedding starts, and/or egg positive samples in the absence of an infection due to coprophagy (Elsemore, 2020). Indeed, lower agreement was observed in older dogs compared to puppies that are more frequently truly infected. Such a disparity was not observed for cats where coprophagy does not occur (Elsemore, 2020).

Currently, the detection of these three nematode species in faeces by the coproantigen ELISAs described above is a service marketed by the company IDEXX and named Faecal Dx™ antigen testing (https://www.idexx.com/en/veterinary/reference-laboratories/fecal-dx-antigen-test/). This service has been used to study the prevalence of canine intestinal parasites in dogs across the United States and Canada (Kotwa et al., 2021; Stafford et al., 2020;

Sweet et al., 2021) and also on a captive wolf population in the United States (Balinsky et al., 2019).

Analysis of the composition of total nematode proteins or the excreted/secreted protein fraction of respective parasite stages offers a great opportunity for developing highly sensitive, specific and low-cost diagnostic methods for the diagnosis of gastrointestinal nematode infections in animals. In particular, the Matrix-assisted laser desorption/ionization-time of flight (MALDI-TOF) mass spectrometry (MS) is a technique which, for example, has become state of the art and routine practice for the diagnosis of many bacterial species (for review, see Feucherolles et al., 2019; Torres-Sangiao et al., 2021). This technique requires only small amounts of protein which is transferred and crystallised on a plate together with an inert matrix, whence the proteins are desorbed and ionised using a laser. The resulting ions are accelerated in an electrical field through a vacuum tube towards the detector which records their charge/mass ratio (m/z) based on the time of flight (TOF). Spectra obtained by this approach are specific for the protein composition of different organisms or tissues and these spectra can be made available in reference databases. However, thus far, only very few studies have been published on the use of this approach in helminthology (using adult helminths) as outlined in a recent review by Feucherolles et al. (2019). The findings of these first studies demonstrate that, also for gastrointestinal nematodes, this technique allows the species-specific detection and differentiation of closely-related species using adult specimens (Bredtmann et al., 2019; Karadjian et al., 2020; Mayer-Scholl et al., 2016; Rivero et al., 2022). This technique also has potential to be of use for the detection of anthelmintic resistance in nematode populations, similar to that described for antibiotic resistance in various bacterial species (for review, see Yoon and Jeong (2021)).

4. Nucleic acid detection methods

4.1 Introduction and background

Methods for the molecular diagnosis of gastrointestinal nematodes (GIN) using nucleic acid detection in livestock and companion animals started to become available during the 1990s after the first gene sequences of parasites such as *H. contortus* had been published. This allowed the development of innovative tools for the detection and identification of, for example, different gastrointestinal strongyle species of ruminants, even at the egg stage. Previously, morphological identification required culturing of eggs to the third larval stage, to allow subsequent microscopic differentiation to the genus level but not for all species to the species level. This procedure does not only take substantially more time (7–8 days for larval culture) than molecular diagnosis but also requires specialised expertise to achieve reliable morphological identification. Also, with regard to species differentiation of adult worms, e.g., following isolation of worms on necropsy, molecular identification is valuable as some species only show slight morphological differences.

In veterinary parasitology, as throughout life sciences, the invention of the Polymerase Chain Reaction method (PCR; Mullis et al., 1986; Saiki et al., 1985, 1988) has to be regarded as a game changer. The well-known key features of PCR-based pathogen detection, such as the very high sensitivity and specificity, as well as technical robustness and widespread accessibility, led to a highly prolific phase of new methods for GIN diagnosis in veterinary medicine being established within only a few years (for review, see Prichard (1997) and Gasser (1999)). Modifications and additional approaches of DNA- or RNA-based parasite detection and characterization such as loop-mediated isothermal amplification (LAMP), randomly amplified polymorphic DNA (RAPD)-PCR or real-time PCR followed and, most recently, high-throughput sequencing technologies, have evolved and are now in widespread use in GIN research as well as for field diagnostics. In parallel with the development of nucleic-acid based diagnostic methods, tests detecting immunological reactions in the host, namely parasite-specific antibodies, have also been introduced. Below, we provide an overview of advances to date in the molecular diagnosis of GIN in veterinary parasitology and also some discussion of currently emerging approaches.

4.2 Sample preparation and extraction of nucleic acids

In most cases of molecular detection of GIN, faecal samples serve as the matrix from which parasites or nucleic acids will be extracted before being amplified and detected. The use of faecal samples or worm stages extracted from faeces for molecular diagnosis is associated with issues arising from (i) the appropriate storage of the faecal sample until further processing, (ii) the successful and efficient extraction of nucleic acids, and (iii) the reliable amplification of these (Azzopardi et al., 2021). During storage of samples, degradation of nucleic acids for example through biological (e.g. by microorganisms) or chemical effects needs to be avoided. While the effects of microorganism-related degradation can at least be significantly reduced by refrigeration or freezing, this is not always feasible depending on the respective field situation. Storage at ambient temperature is considerably less effort and thus different preservatives allowing for medium to long-term storage without cooling/freezing have been tested in this context. However, not all preservatives are similarly well suited for this purpose as, for example, Harmon et al. (2007a) showed that the use of formalin results in degradation of nucleic acids, whereas Lugol's iodine and sodium azide do not, when used for the detection of *H. contortus* from sheep faecal samples. The DNA amplification of four different soil-transmitted-helminth species using human stool samples stored over up to 425 days at 4 °C either in ethanol, potassium dichloride and RNAlater showed these storage conditions to be stable (Ayana et al., 2019).

For the extraction of nucleic acids from GIN, the parasite stages have to be lysed, which can be achieved by freezing and thawing and/or by mechanical means such as bead-beating. While the latter has been described to be of advantage particularly for DNA extraction from thick-shelled nematode eggs such as *Ascaris* spp. (Amoah et al., 2020) and, in particular, *Trichuris* spp. (Demeler et al., 2013b), repeated boiling and freezing cycles were found to be sufficient when using, for example, human and ruminant strongyle species as well as the ascarids *Toxocara* spp. (Demeler et al., 2013b). Following parasite lysis, amplification of nucleic acids can effectively be done directly and with sensitivities as low as a few eggs for different human and animal intestinal nematode species (Demeler et al., 2013b). Alternatively, nucleic acids may be extracted prior to amplification and several commercial kits have been employed and compared for this purpose, resulting in significantly different sensitivities depending on the particular kit used (e.g. Amoah et al., 2020; Ayana et al., 2019).

In this context, it is relevant to address the presence of biotic components in the faeces, such as PCR-inhibitors from faecal samples like bilirubin, bile salt or phytic acids, which can negatively impact the outcome of the molecular method used (Sidstedt et al., 2020). PCR inhibitors may influence the molecular detection process in multiple ways including interference with the cell lysis step, inactivation of the enzyme used for nucleic acid amplification or by binding to the nucleic acids, thus preventing enzyme access (for review, see Rådström et al., 2004). However, through genetic engineering, such as the addition of a non-specific DNA-binding protein domain and the processivity of PCR-polymerases, the effect of inhibitors can be significantly reduced (Wang et al., 2004). Also, diluting the respective DNA sample can result in a reduction of PCR inhibition (Demeler et al., 2013b).

During real-time PCR, inhibitors may also interfere with efficient fluorescence detection. Specific PCR buffers have also been developed to overcome PCR inhibitor effects (for review, see Sidstedt et al. (2020)).

4.3 Conventional PCR methods

4.3.1 Conventional PCR methods for the detection of GIN

For the molecular identification of GIN, a range of different DNA or RNA target sequences, such as β-tubulin or ribosomal RNA genes, have been employed in PCR assays, allowing species-specific and sensitive (as low as a single egg) detection of free-living parasite stages (for review, see Gasser, 1999; Prichard, 1997). In particular, ribosomal RNA gene sequences such as the internal transcribed spacers (ITS) provide features which make them most valuable as targets for high sensitivity and species-specific detection. They are tandemly arrayed in many repeats (often more than a hundred) and have evolved in a pattern of 'concerted evolution', which means that they exhibit greater within—than between-species similarity (see Gasser, 1999). Numerous PCR-assays have been developed based mostly on the second internal transcribed spacer (ITS2) sequences, for example, of ruminant strongyle species. By employing PCR primer sequences which result in amplification of fragments with different lengths for different worm species, even semi-quantitative species-specific detection protocols were described in the early days of PCR diagnostics (Zarlenga et al., 1998a). Because rRNA gene sequences such as ITS do show some level of within-species sequence heterogeneity, the more rapidly and less conserved mitochondrial DNA sequences have been found to be more suitable for studying population structure and the phylogenetic analysis of closely related species (Ramünke et al., 2018; Zarlenga et al., 1998b). Mitochondrial DNA sequences employed for genetic diversity and population structure analysis include cytochrome *c* oxidase subunit I (COI), NADH dehydrogenase subunit 4 (NAD4) or 16S rRNA genes (Brasil et al., 2012; Campbell et al., 2008; Hussain et al., 2014; Pitaksakulrat et al., 2021; Ramünke et al., 2018).

By post-amplification processing of PCR fragments, an additional level of analytical power can be obtained. For example, PCR-restriction fragment length polymorphism (PCR-RFLP), i.e., the digestion of PCR products with endonucleases, which cut at a specific nucleotide sequence of, e.g., four base pairs, can be used to obtain fragments with species—or even strain-specific length patterns. This is an efficient, comparatively low-tech and inexpensive approach, and so numerous studies and protocols have been described for the detection and differentiation of GIN (e.g. Gasser et al., 1994; Gasser and Hoste, 1995; Meshgi et al., 2015; Newton et al., 1998; Patrelle et al., 2014; Wang et al., 2012a; Zhao et al., 2015).

A broad range of PCR-based DNA-fingerprinting methods allowing the differentiation of different populations of GIN, both within and between species, have been developed, including RAPD (Humbert and Cabaret, 1995), microsatellite analysis, amplified fragment length polymorphism (AFLP; (Troell et al., 2006)) or representational difference analysis (RDA) for ruminant GIN (for review, see Gasser (1999)). While some of these methods have become less frequently used in more recent published studies, the examination of population structure by microsatellite analysis continues to be reported in numerous publications such as Sargison et al. (2019b), George et al. (2021), Chaudhry et al. (2020) or Portanier et al. (2019). Despite the increasing availability and reduced costs of the continuously developing next-generation-sequencing opportunities, microsatellite analysis obviously still proves to be of some value, presumably because of its high resolution and precision. One illustrative example is the analysis of reduced genetic diversity during the generation of *H. contortus* inbred lines (Sargison et al., 2018). Micro- or minisatellites consist of short tandem nucleotide epeats (e.g. CA or GA) which exist in all eukaryotes and are randomly dispersed in mostly non-coding regions of the genome. As such they tend to accumulate mutations by insertions/deletions, which is a meaningful feature when analysing genetic processes in populations. For example, microsatellite markers have been developed for the ruminant GIN such as *H. contortus* (Hoekstra et al., 1997; Redman et al., 2015; Santos et al., 2017) *Teladorsagia* spp. (Grillo et al., 2006; Redman et al., 2015) and *Trichostrongylus* spp. (Temperley et al., 2009; Redman et al., 2015). One of the prerequisites in using this approach is the necessity first to identify and characterise suitable microsatellite markers for the respective organism. This has been done initially by screening DNA libraries with radioactively labelled oligonucleotide probes (e.g. $(CA)_{25}$) and subsequent sequencing of up- and downstream regions to identify microsatellites with appropriate length as well as the flanking sequences, allowing the design of suitable PCR primers for specific amplification (Hoekstra et al., 1997). Finally, each microsatellite marker candidate has to be checked for length polymorphisms and, when used for population structure analysis, multiple markers distributed through the genome are required. Thus, the complete process is rather time and effort demanding. Furthermore, although in principle cross-species use of microsatellites has been described for ruminant GIN, it is apparently only feasible to a much lesser extent than in other groups of organisms (Grillo et al., 2008; Papaiakovou et al., 2022; Temperley et al., 2009).

4.3.2 Conventional PCR methods for the detection of anthelmintic resistance

For the molecular detection of anthelmintic resistance (AR), a basic understanding of the underlying resistance-associated genetic changes is required, including for example, the question: "only single or multiple changes occur in the respective nematode species?" This information is in principle available for the benzimidazole drug class, where it was initially shown for *H. contortus* that specific single-nucleotide-polymorphisms (SNPs) in the isotype 1 β-tubulin gene at codons 200 (Kwa et al., 1995), 167 (Silvestre and Cabaret, 2002) and 198 (Ghisi et al., 2007) are associated with resistance. In due course, respective allele-specific PCRs for the detection of these resistance-associated alleles were developed (for review, see (Humbert et al., 2001; von Samson-Himmelstjerna, 2006). Recent reviews have covered the subject of conventional PCR methods for AR detection (Kotze et al., 2014, 2020).

Conventional PCR methods allowed the genotyping of nematode stages and thus the assessment of the respective composition of worm populations by analysing representative numbers of individual worm DNA samples. However, as this approach requires considerable time and costs, subsequent efforts were directed at the development of tools allowing the analysis of pooled samples (see below).

4.4 Real-time PCR approaches

4.4.1 Single-plex PCR approaches

Real-time PCRs were developed not only to identify positive samples but also to obtain quantitative data. Based on ITS-2 sequences, such PCRs have been described for trichostrongyloid parasites of ruminants (von Samson-Himmelstjerna et al., 2002; Harmon et al., 2007b; Learmount et al., 2009), for *S. vulgaris* in horses (Nielsen et al., 2012, 2008), and *A. suum* in pigs (Pecson et al., 2006), as well as for human parasites such as *Necator americanus* hookworms (Wang et al., 2012a,b). Sensitivity can be further improved by targeting non-coding, highly repetitive (typically >1000 copies per haploid genome) DNA sequences in the genome as described for *A. suum* and the human pathogens *N. americanus*,

Ancylostoma duodenale, *Trichuris trichiura*, *A. lumbricoides*, and *S. stercoralis* (Pilotte et al., 2016, 2019). The latter approach was also used to develop a specific real-time PCR detection method for the zoonotic hookworm *Ancylostoma ceylanicum*, which shows considerable similarity in the ITS2 region to other members of the genus *Ancylostoma* (Papaiakovou et al., 2017).

Detection of eggs of human or zoonotic soil transmitted nematodes in soil samples and waste-water is routinely investigated using real-time PCR. In this context, it is important to discriminate between viable and dead eggs. The simplest approach in this direction has been applied to eggs of *A. suum* to determine the effect of inactivation procedures such as heat treatment, UV light or exposure to disinfectants on egg viability. For this purpose, homogenous, undeveloped *A. suum* egg samples were exposed to inactivation conditions and then allowed to develop for up to 30 days. Then, a real-time PCR targeting the ITS-1 region was applied to compare the signals between control eggs that had developed normally and inactivated eggs, the latter showing increased DNA content following continued cell division (Pecson et al., 2006). Results were comparable with microscopic discrimination of undeveloped and embryonated eggs. However, the approach is obviously not well suited for analysing egg populations that contain eggs of various ages, and thus developmental stages, and therefore can only rarely be applied directly to the analysis of soil or wastewater samples. Ethidium monoazide and propidium monoazide (PMA) have been used to destroy DNA from the environment and in non-viable cells (Fittipaldi et al., 2011; Taskin et al., 2011). The DNA intercalating dyes bind to the DNA and can then be activated by light to react with the DNA. The PMA approach has also been used to determine the fraction of viable eggs of *Ascaris* spp. (Acosta Soto et al., 2017; Gyawali et al., 2016; Ravindran et al., 2019) and human and zoonotic hookworms (Gyawali et al., 2015, 2016, 2017) by comparing the results of PMA-qPCR with simple qPCR.

Real-time PCRs have also been used to quantify allele frequencies for isotype 1 β-tubulin genes. Polymorphisms in codons 167 (F167Y), 198 (E198A and others) and 200 (F200Y) have been implicated in resistance of strongyle nematodes against benzimidazoles. Such assays have predominantly focused on codon 200 and have been described for cyathostomines (von Samson-Himmelstjerna et al., 2003), *H. contortus* (Walsh et al., 2007) and several hookworm species (Schwenkenbecher et al., 2007; Schwenkenbecher and Kaplan, 2009). However, real-time PCR quickly proved to be inferior in comparison with pyrosequencing (von Samson-Himmelstjerna et al., 2009) and has never been used for larger epidemiological surveys.

Real-time PCR was shown to be an excellent tool to quantify the amount of a specific DNA in a sample (Nielsen et al., 2008, 2012; Pilotte et al., 2019; von Samson-Himmelstjerna et al., 2002; Wang et al., 2012b) but difficulties due to the potential presence of PCR inhibitors in faecal samples have also been noted (Harmon et al., 2007b). Presence of inhibitors can be overcome using particular DNA extraction methods such as those in commercial kits for extraction of DNA from inhibitor-rich matrices or inhibitor-resistant polymerases, as detailed above (see Section 4.2). To make sure that amplification is not completely inhibited in such samples, amplification of a control DNA fragment is included. This can either be derived from host DNA or a pan-nematode PCR can be used as control if the real-time PCR aims to detect or quantify a particular parasite species in a mixed infection (e.g. *S. vulgaris* in the presence of a large variety of cyathostomin eggs) (Gehlen et al., 2020). However, such internal standards also have limitations since host DNA in faecal samples might be degraded to various extents and the amount of the standard might be extremely high compared with the amount of DNA for the pathogen species of interest. Under these circumstances, the successful amplification of the standard allows only limited conclusions about the chances of amplifying DNA of the target pathogen. An alternative approach is the use of an external standard that can, e.g., be added to the lysis buffer before DNA extraction. DNA of DNA viruses with sufficiently large genomes such as phocine herpes virus DNA can be used for this purpose since this will co-purify with the host and pathogen DNA in the samples (Niesters, 2004; Verweij et al., 2009). Such external standards and comparison of the signals from external standard and target species allow determination of copy number of the target DNA per volume of the original sample.

However, there are also general problems using qPCR approaches for quantification of parasite stages. Apart from the fact that the number of eggs does not necessarily correlate with the number of adult worms and can, for example, fluctuate highly from day to day, even within an individual host, as described for several Ostertaginae such as *T. circumcincta*, whereas some strongyle species such as *Haemonchus* spp. and *Chabertia* spp. show quite constant egg output per female (Gasser et al., 2008). Eggs, and in particular larvae, of different species contain different numbers of cells and thus genome copies and a single genome may contain a different number of copies of the target sequence if multi-copy targets such as rRNA or repetitive elements are used. Therefore, it is not sufficient to show linearity of real-time PCR signals over a wide range of template concentrations but also to calibrate signals using the relevant stages of the parasites (e.g. eggs, first or third stage larvae). This is even more relevant—and technically complex—if the aim is to determine the proportion of all parasite species in a multi-species infection.

4.4.2 Detection of multiple nematode species using a single primer pair

Primer pairs that are able to amplify corresponding but variable regions from multiple related nematode species have been widely used and the above-mentioned ITS-2 and ITS-1 regions are the most widely used of such target regions. Additional targets flanked by conserved primer binding sites are hypervariable regions in the 18S (small subunit) and 28S (large subunit) rRNA genes and the external transcribed spacers. This well-established strategy employed in conventional PCR could certainly be developed further by discriminating the different PCR products directly in the PCR tube instead of using approaches such as RFLP or Sanger sequencing. In principle, there are two different approaches available to achieve this goal, i.e., using a mixture of different species-specific probes coupled to different fluorophores or an analysis of the PCR product after completion of the exponential phase of the PCR using a high-resolution melt (HRM) analysis. The approach using species-specific probes has been successfully used to discriminate larvae of the filarial parasites *Onchocerca volvulus* and *Onchocerca lupi* from human samples (Acosta Soto et al., 2017), but this strategy has not been used for GIN to the knowledge of the authors. However, McNally et al. (2013) used a very similar approach, that is discussed in more detail in Section 4.4.3. The same principle has also been very successfully applied for droplet digital PCR (ddPCR) (see Section 4.5.1).

High-resolution melt (HMR) PCR is basically a real-time PCR using a fluorescent dye that specifically binds double-stranded DNA and that strongly increases its fluorescence upon DNA binding (Wittwer et al., 2003). For the purpose of HRM, dyes are required that can be used in concentrations allowing complete saturation of available DNA binding sites without inhibition of the PCR. Dyes suitable for this purpose are LCGreen Plus, SYTO 9 and EvaGreen among others (Wittwer, 2009). Using slow denaturation of the PCR product after the final amplification cycle leads to gradual denaturation of the double-stranded DNA. The melting temperature, defined as the temperature at which half of the DNA is denatured, depends on the composition and the length of the DNA when under constant chemical conditions; in particular, concentrations of mono- and divalent cations and organic components such as the PCR enhancers DMSO and betaine also affect the melting temperature. In addition, local effects such as variation of the GC content along the length of the DNA molecule and stacking, i.e., direct interaction of adjacent aromatic rings of bases, lead to the phenomenon that melting of double strands can occur in some parts of the molecule earlier than in others (Wittwer et al., 2003). These phenomena can be exploited by recording fluorescence intensity continuously while samples are slowly heated to 94 °C. If melting occurs simultaneously along the whole amplicon, simple melting curves with a single peak in the first derivative ($dF/d\vartheta$) of the melting curve are observed. However, when domains with distinct melting properties occur in the amplicon, melting curves can be more complicated and exhibit two or even more melting peaks (Wittwer et al., 2003). Pan-nematode primer pairs such as a 28S rRNA primer pair flanking a hypervariable loop or ITS-2 primers have been used before to discriminate *Toxocara* spp. and human hookworms, respectively (Demeler et al., 2013b). However, neither method is widely applicable since the 28S primer pair is pan-nematode and, e.g., in dogs, it might not only amplify *T. canis* and *T. cati* (shed after coprophagy) but also *Toxascaris leonina*, *A. caninum*, *A. ceylanicum*, *Uncinaria stenocephala*, *S. stercoralis* and *T. vulpis*. If so many different pathogens have to be considered and might also occur as multi-species co-infections, it is unlikely that any methodology could be established to identify all of them unequivocally. For the ITS-2 primer pair, the situation is highly dependent on the host species. The primer pair is specific for strongyles although DNA from non-parasitic clade V nematodes is presumably also amplified. The use of ITS-2 amplicons for sheep samples cannot be expected to be informative since more than 10 different species are known to occur in sheep populations (Zajac and Garza, 2020). In contrast, in dogs, only amplification of hookworms (*A. caninum*, *U. stenocephala*, depending on the geographical region also *A. ceylanicum* or *A. braziliense*) and lungworms is to be expected. Thus, if purified eggs are used as the template, the ITS-2 might be well suited to discriminate between local hookworm species using HRM analysis of the ITS-2 products. However, melting curves of hookworm ITS-2 amplicons are complex with three peaks occurring in *A. caninum* (Demeler et al., 2013b). High-resolution melt PCR targeting the ITS-2 has indeed been used to discriminate between five species of hookworm transmitted between humans (*A. duodenale*, *N. americanus*) or infecting humans as accidental hosts (zoonotic species *A. ceylanicum*, *A. caninum*, *A. braziliense*) (Ngui et al., 2012). The method uses primers not targeting the highly conserved regions flanking the ITS-2 but degenerated primers specific for hookworm ITS-2 sequences. With this approach the authors aim to exclude amplification of other clade V nematodes that are occasionally found in humans such as *T. colubriformis* and *Oesophagostomum* spp. High-resolution melt PCR has also been applied to discriminate between feline hookworms *A. tubaeformae* and *A. ceylanicum* (Fu et al., 2019) and differentiate eggs of *Spirocerca lupi* from those of other nematodes in dogs (Rojas et al., 2017). Recently, a similar approach was used to identify samples positive for *Strongylus equinus*, *Strongylus edentatus* or *Strongylus asini* and discriminate between these large strongyle species according to their melting curves (Jürgenschellert et al., 2022).

In addition to analyses of melting of the complete amplicon, several variants have been described that use hybridisation of short, unlabelled probes (see Erali et al. (2008) for review). Snap-back primers include the probe attached at the 5′-end of the primer. This probe is complementary to a region of the amplicon immediately downstream of the primer. This allows the primer to fold back to the template, forming a hairpin loop. Using an asymmetric PCR approach with a higher concentration of the snapback primer than the second primer, a mixture of double-stranded amplicons and single-stranded products with the hairpin on one end are formed. In the short double-stranded stem of the hairpin, mismatches have stronger effects and this increases the power to discriminate different sequence variants (Zhou et al., 2008). This approach has been used to discriminate the three sympatric *Haemonchus* species *H. contortus*, *Haemonchus placei* and *Haemonchus longistipes* based on polymorphisms in their ITS-2 sequences (Pichler et al., 2017). The melting curves of the snapback stem loop product were shown to discriminate the three species more reliably than the melting curves of the full-length amplicon. However, it should be kept in mind that species diagnosis based on SNPs is risky, since polymorphisms that are considered to be fixed between species may turn out to occur in both species once a larger number of sequences from different populations of the species becomes available, as discussed previously for *Cooperia* spp. (Ramünke et al., 2018).

4.4.3 Multiplex PCR approaches

Multiplexing multiple PCRs in a single tube is attractive since it reduces the amount of hands-on time and total time required to detect multiple parasites in the same sample. Using species-specific primers and probes with fluorescent labels in different colours, real-time PCR is ideally suited for multiplexing since many modern real-time PCR cyclers offer channels in multiple parts of the optical spectrum. It is obviously desirable to combine detection of GIN in faecal samples with detection of other pathogens shed in the faeces and sharing similar routes of transmission (for epidemiological studies) or sharing similar clinical symptoms (to rapidly evaluate multiple differential diagnostic options). Although all of the PCRs mentioned in the following section are conducted as real-time PCRs, their major aim is to identify positive samples and not to quantify egg shedding intensity.

In human tropical medicine, multiplex PCR assays targeting parasitic nematodes using phocine herpesvirus added to the lysis buffer as control have been developed and expanded since the first application by Verweij et al. (2007) to diagnose the hookworms *A. duodenale* and *N. americanus* and the nodular worm *Oesophagostomum bifurcum*. The method was further adapted to include *A. lumbricoides* and *S. stercoralis* while removing the *O. bifurcum* PCR from the protocol (Basuni et al., 2011, 2012; Taniuchi et al., 2011; Gordon et al., 2015). Llewellyn et al. (2016) developed a pentaplex PCR targeting the GINs *Ancylostoma* spp., *N. americanus*, *Ascaris* spp. and *T. trichiura* with equine herpes virus as the positive control. A multiplex PCR detecting *A. lumbricoides*, *A. duodenale*, *N. americanus*, *S. stercoralis* and *T. trichiura* together with three protozoan parasites (*Giardia duodenalis*, *Cryptosporidium parvum/hominis* and *Entamoeba histolytica*) has also been described (Mejia et al., 2013; Cimino et al., 2015).

The number of publications describing multiplex real-time PCRs for parasites of domestic animals is considerably smaller. For the sheep parasites *H. contortus*, *T. circumcincta* and *Trichostrongylus* spp., McNally et al. (2013) used an approach employing a common reverse primer (the NC2 primer widely used for strongyle ITS-2 PCRs (Gasser et al., 1993)) combined with almost identical forward primers and genus-specific hydrolyzation (TaqMan) probes. The assays showed excellent correlation with FECs of sheep faeces spiked with eggs from individual species (McNally et al., 2013). The authors noticed considerable inhibition of the PCR despite inclusion of an absorption of tannins using polyvinylpolypyrrolidone that could be mostly overcome by dilution of the DNA 1:8-fold or more. Reslova et al. (2021) recently described two multiplex PCRs for the detection of *H. contortus*, *T. circumcincta* and *T. colubriformis* in the first and *Nematodirus battus*, *Ashworthius sidemi* and *Chabertia ovina* in the second multiplex PCR. Both PCRs contained template and primers/probes for the same internal amplification control to detect potential PCR inhibition and a commercial kit for isolation of DNA from faecal samples was used to remove all potential PCR inhibitors. The authors also observed high specificity of their PCRs towards other species occurring in sheep faeces such as *Cooperia* spp. and *Oesophagostomum columbianum*. Finally, the authors developed a calibration curve to translate Cq to EPG values (Reslova et al., 2021). Two multiplex PCR assays have also been described for the detection of the complete spectrum of zoonotic canine hookworm species (Massetti et al., 2020). The authors also used a commercial DNA isolation kit, removing PCR inhibitors. The first multiplex PCR contained a common primer pair for *A. caninum* and *A. ceylanicum* and discriminates the species using different TaqMan probes while the second multiplex PCR used the same approach for *A. brazilienze* and *U. stenocephala.* Both PCRs also contained primers and probes to detect mammalian (canine) host DNA and equine herpes virus 4 (EHP4) (internal amplification control) (Massetti et al., 2020). In contrast to the use of viral DNA as an extraction control (described above for diagnostic PCRs targeting human parasites), the EHP4 DNA in this case was only added to the master mix and was not already in the extraction buffer. This PCR was successfully applied in epidemiological studies on zoonotic helminths in Nigeria (Kamani et al., 2021; Massetti et al., 2021).

4.4.4 PCR approaches to estimate multi-species equivalents of faecal egg counts

Most of the real-time PCRs described thus far aimed to answer the simple diagnostic question of whether a particular parasite is present or not in a sample or to provide an estimate of the intensity of egg shedding for one or a few parasite species. To obtain molecular data that can replace EPG counting methods and are specific for individual parasite species or at least genera, quantitative real-time PCRs are required for all the relevant parasite species occurring in a particular host, and all need to be assessed quantitatively using samples with defined epg and not only using DNA standards with defined copy numbers. Bott et al. (2009) approached this aim by establishing individual real-time PCRs for the sheep parasites *H. contortus, T. circumcincta, Trichostrongylus* spp., *C. oncophora, C. ovina, O. columbianum* and *Oesophagostomum venulosum* using species-specific forward primers and NC2 as the common reverse primer. DNA was isolated from eggs purified using flotation and diluted to prevent PCR inhibition. PCR products were detected using the double-stranded DNA specific dye SYTO 9 and specificity of the amplification products was evaluated using melting curve analyses. The authors also determined the EPG microscopically and aimed to combine molecular and microscopical data to monitor presence of parasites and estimate egg count reduction after anthelmintic treatment at the species level (Bott et al., 2009). The method was then used to determine prevalence of these parasitic nematodes and their contribution to egg shedding in south-eastern Australia (Roeber et al., 2011).

Furthermore, the authors were able to extend this method to conduct a PCR-coupled FECRT to identify the nematode species resistant to anthelmintics (Roeber et al., 2012b). An automated method that appears to be built on this approach is used in the multiplexed-tandem (MT-)PCR system developed by AusDiagnostics (Sydney, Australia). The MT-PCR approach uses a first amplification phase to enrich the target using a low number of PCR cycles followed by analytical amplification with species-specific primers (Stanley and Szewczuk, 2005). Before the second phase, PCR products of the first phase are diluted and reamplified. The MT-PCR assay for sheep strongyle nematodes by Roeber et al. (2012a) targets the same parasitic nematode species as established before (Bott et al., 2009; Roeber et al., 2011) but information on whether the analytical PCRs use the same primers is not available. Automated handling of samples using a robotic platform decreases hands-on time and increases precision. The MT-PCR was shown to be highly sensitive and specific using both Australian and European sheep samples (Roeber et al., 2012a, 2017b). There was also good agreement with the results of larval cultures followed by morphological species identification. A cattle version of this assay targeted the genera *Cooperia*, *Ostertagia*, *Haemonchus*, *Trichostrongylus*, *Oesophagostomum*, *Bunostomum*, *Dictyocaulus* and also included a pan-nematode primer pair. It was also reported to have sensitivities and specificities >90% (Roeber et al., 2017a). Furthermore, the method has been used for diagnosis of the major human soil-transmitted helminths (*A. lumbricoides*, *A. duodenale*, *A. ceylanicum*, *N. americanus* and *T. trichiura*) (Stracke et al., 2019). None of the aforementioned MT-PCRs targeting GIN of animals or humans is listed among the available assays on the AusDiagnostics webpage (last visited 18.04.2022).

4.5 Droplet digital PCR

4.5.1 Droplet digital PCR for nematode species diagnosis

Droplet digital PCR (ddPCR) combines probe-based PCR (typically TaqMan probes) with a microfluidics analysis platform. In contrast to real-time PCR, ddPCR relies on analysis of the endpoint of the PCR reaction. Basically, the PCR reaction is subdivided into thousands of small partitions (droplets) by a variety of different available methods. These droplets ideally contain only a single or no template DNA molecule (Chen et al., 2021). After PCR, the number of fluorescent droplets is counted using specialised reader instruments. This offers the possibility to determine the number of template molecules by counting the number of droplets with a particular fluorescence and without the need for standard curves (Chen et al., 2021).

Of course, the situation is more complicated in the real world and droplets with more than one template molecule do occur and this is compensated for by mathematical modelling applying Poisson distribution models (Li et al., 2018). Applying a single primer pair with a single fluorescent probe, Yu et al. (2020) demonstrated that ddPCR was more sensitive than real-time PCR for the detection of *Trichuris* spp. in sheep. When the template copy number was low, the proportion of positive assays was significantly higher than with qPCR. Similar observations were reported for the detection of human infections with *S. stercoralis* (Iamrod et al., 2022). The ddPCR approach has advantages when used for the simultaneous detection of multiple pathogens. The simple counting method to obtain quantitative data means that a direct comparison between multiple species targeted in a single assay is possible and this does not rely directly on factors such as PCR efficacy. Using genus-specific primers and probe sets, Tarbiat et al. (2021) were able to detect individual and co-infections of chicken with *Ascaridia galli* and *Heterakis gallinarum* in faecal samples. Very low copy numbers of one parasite could be reliably detected in the presence of a high abundance of the other. For the cattle parasites *O. ostertagi* and *C. oncophora*, Baltrušis et al. (2019) used a single primer pair to amplify partial ITS-2 fragments from both parasites and combined this PCR with two probes specific for each of the parasites as well as a universal probe. This assay was able to detect *C. oncophora* DNA when it represented only 2.5% of the template and *O. ostertagi* even when it was present as only 0.67% of the total template. For sheep parasites, the three major pathogenic GIN genera *Haemonchus*, *Teladorsagia* and *Trichostrongylus* were targeted in an equivalent assay using genus-specific probes (Elmahalawy et al., 2018). This assay was able to substitute a conventional FECRT using the universal probe and also to obtain corresponding reduction values for larvae from each of the three target genera. The assay has been further used to investigate the effects of nematode infections on activity patterns of sheep (Högberg et al., 2021) and of lambing season of ewes on GIN egg shedding (Höglund et al., 2021).

4.5.2 Droplet digital PCR vs pyrosequencing for quantification of SNPs associated with benzimidazole resistance

Another highly relevant application of ddPCR is the quantification of SNPs in the isotype 1 β-tubulin genes of strongyle nematodes. With regard to parasitic nematodes, pyrosequencing was first used for genotyping *H. contortus* populations according to two SNPs in the ITS-1 sequence (Troell et al., 2003). Since pyrosequencing has been shown to be superior to real-time

PCR for quantification of SNPs in codon 200 of the isotype 1 β-tubulin gene (von Samson-Himmelstjerna et al., 2009), it has become the method of choice for quantification of benzimidazole resistance associated SNPs in strongyle nematodes. Methods have been published for codons 167, 198 and 200 of many parasitic nematodes such as *Haemonchus* spp. (Ademola et al., 2015; von Samson-Himmelstjerna et al., 2009), *T. circumcincta* (Martínez-Valladares et al., 2012), *C. oncophora* (Demeler et al., 2013a), *O. ostertagi* (Demeler et al., 2013a), *Trichostrongylus* spp. (Ramünke et al., 2016), *Nematodirus battus* (Melville et al., 2020), *S. vulgaris* (Jürgenschellert et al., 2022) and the human parasites *N. americanus* (Gandasegui et al., 2021), *A. lumbricoides* and *T. trichiura* (Diawara et al., 2009). Pyrosequencing has been used for many epidemiological surveys (Ademola et al., 2015; Barrere et al., 2013; Chaudhry et al., 2014, 2015a,b; Diawara et al., 2009; Fávero et al., 2020; Hinney et al., 2020; Martínez-Valladares et al., 2012; Melville et al., 2020; Mohammedsalih et al., 2020, 2021; Ramünke et al., 2016; Skuce et al., 2010). However, the method also has its limitations since low amounts of PCR products lead to unreliable signals (see Mohammedsalih et al., 2020) and thus many of the aforementioned studies have only considered frequencies of resistant SNPs above 10% as reliable. More importantly, some kinds of polymorphisms cannot be analysed by pyrosequencing at all, for instance, presence of two SNPs at consecutive positions can be impossible to analyse. Regarding SNPs associated with benzimidazole resistance in the isotype 1 β-tubulin, this is particularly problematic for the reported polymorphism E198L (GAA ≥ TTA) that has been found in recent years in *T. circumcincta* in the United Kingdom, Ireland and Spain, *Trichostronglylus* spp. in North America and in *H. contortus* in Sweden and Sudan (Avramenko et al., 2019; Baltrušis et al., 2018; Keegan et al., 2017; Martínez-Valladares et al., 2020; Mohammedsalih et al., 2020, 2021; Redman et al., 2015, 2019).

The ddPCR method has only recently been used for the quantification of SNPs in the isotype 1 β-tubulin gene of a single parasitic nematode, *H. contortus*. Assays for the most common polymorphisms F200Y and F167Y have been published (Baltrušis et al., 2018, 2020). For the exchange in codon 200, an excellent correlation between ddPCR and PacBio-based deep amplicon sequencing was observed (Baltrušis et al., 2018). The limit of detection for the mutant sequence variant in codon 200 was as low as 2.6% for ddPCR. The ddPCR assays for codons 167 and 200 were further compared with pyrosequencing assays showing good agreement (Baltrušis et al., 2020). Both assays were applied to field samples collected from sheep in

Sweden, showing that the mutation in codon 200 was much more frequent than the codon 167 mutation (Baltrušis et al., 2020). Hinney et al. (2021) reported the development of ddPCR assays for detection of all four major polymorphisms in the isotype I β-tubulin gene of *H. contortus*, i.e., F167Y, E198A, E98L and F200Y.

4.6 Isothermal amplification

Isothermal amplification techniques have the advantage that less sophisticated equipment is required in comparison with PCR which requires rapid and exact changes of temperatures (Tröger et al., 2015). Isothermal amplification protocols have often been reported to be at least as sensitive or even more sensitive than PCR (Wong et al., 2018). In its simplest form, isothermal amplification can be successful using a conventional water bath. Since isothermal amplification protocols cannot use DNA denaturation by heating to temperatures above 90 °C, DNA polymerases with strong strand displacement activity but lacking a 5′ to >3′ exonuclease activity are required. The prototype example of such an enzyme is the large fragment of *Bst* DNA polymerase, although other polymerases have also been used in isothermal amplification (Tröger et al., 2015). In contrast to Taq DNA polymerase, such a polymerase will not degrade the DNA strand in front of the primer—as happens during hydrolysis of TaqMan probes—but will displace the strand and replace it with a newly synthesised strand. Efficient primer binding requires the presence of single stranded loops in the amplification products since displacement of long double-stranded products by short primers is obviously unfavourable if both show 100% identity. Isothermal amplification processes have been suggested to be useful for pen-side or point-of care diagnosis. For pen-side or point-of-care application, read-out devices based on smartphone cameras have been developed (Chen et al., 2017; Ganguli et al., 2017; Heithoff et al., 2022).

The most widely used isothermal amplification method is loop-mediated isothermal amplification (LAMP) (Wong et al., 2018), which typically uses the large fragment of the *Bst* polymerase. One of the advantages of LAMP is its robustness regarding the presence of compounds that are potent inhibitors of PCR (Francois et al., 2011). This allows the use of biological matrices such as blood, nematode eggs or crude faecal extracts or urine without applying elaborate and expensive DNA purification protocols (Francois et al., 2011).

Protocols for diagnosis of GIN have been published among others for *H. contortus* in small ruminants (Khangembam et al., 2021; Ljungström et al., 2018; Melville et al., 2014; Yang et al., 2017), *Toxocara* spp. in cats, dogs and soil samples (Avila et al., 2021b; Azimian et al., 2021; Kazemi et al., 2020; Khoshakhlagh et al., 2017; Macuhova et al., 2010),

A. caninum in dog faeces (Avila et al., 2021a), *N. americanus* (Mugambi et al., 2015), *A. lumbricoides* (Shiraho et al., 2016), *T. trichiura* (Ngari et al., 2020), *S. stercoralis* (Fernández-Soto et al., 2020; Watts et al., 2014, 2018) in human faecal and urine samples. Despite the fact that pen-side detection can be achieved with lateral-flow devices using LAMP (Khangembam et al., 2021; Wong et al., 2018), no commercialised tests for any GIN of veterinary importance are available to the knowledge of the authors. This is in contrast to human protozoan parasites such as *Plasmodium* spp. (González et al., 2012; Antinori et al., 2021).

SmartAmp 2 is an isothermal amplification process similar to LAMP that also uses primer binding to loop regions and the *Aac* DNA polymerase with strand displacement activity (Baum et al., 2005). For species diagnosis of human soil-transmitted helminth, colorimetric and fluorescent real-time SmartAmp2 assays have been developed to specifically detect *N. americanus*, *A. lumbricoides* and *T. trichiura* in crude lysates of eggs or larvae (Rashwan et al., 2017a). SmartAmp 2 can be conducted in the presence of the protein TaqMutS, which has the property to bind to positions in double-stranded DNA carrying mismatches (Mitani et al., 2007). This completely prevents amplification from primers carrying a single mismatch and is thus highly suitable for the detection of SNPs. In the context of benzimidazole resistance, SmartAmp 2 assays for the isotype 1 β-tubulin gene of *N. americanus* targeting the polymorphisms F167Y, E198E and F200Y have been described (Rashwan et al., 2016). These assays were validated using purified DNA and crude lysates and Rashwan et al. (2016) were able to demonstrate allele-specific amplification from pools as well as from individual eggs or larvae. Using artificial mixtures of plasmids containing the target sequences, as little as 1% of the resistance-associated alleles could be reliably detected in 99% of the wild-type allele (Rashwan et al., 2016). Similar assays were established for all three polymorphisms for the only β-tubulin gene encoded in the *T. trichiura* genome and for the bt-A β-tubulin gene from *A. lumbricoides* (Rashwan et al., 2017b). However, the latter is only one out of eight β-tubulin paralogs in the *A. lumbricoides* genome (Roose et al., 2021) and this isotype is probably not involved in benzimidazole resistance in ascarids (Martin et al., 2021; Özben et al., 2022; Roose et al., 2021).

4.7 DNA-sequencing approaches

4.7.1 Molecular barcoding for nematode species identification using 1st generation sequencing

DNA sequencing has been used in parasite diagnostics for almost 30 years. It has been used predominantly to determine the identity of parasitic nematode specimens using an appropriate taxonomic marker and is often described as DNA barcoding (Gasser et al., 1993; Lichtenfels et al., 1997; Oliveira-Arbex et al., 2016; Zarlenga et al., 1994; Zhu et al., 1998).

Species identification of parasitic nematodes using morphological criteria not only requires substantial expertise but can be unreliable when applied to closely related species using eggs and larval stages, and often only reliably discriminates to the genus level (Dorris et al., 1999; Gasser et al., 2008; Seesao et al., 2017). Consequently, DNA sequencing has been used to confirm the species identity of adult nematodes collected from necropsies or from eggs and larvae extracted from faeces of livestock and companion animals, both in research and in routine diagnostics (Gasser et al., 1993; Lichtenfels et al., 1997; Oliveira-Arbex et al., 2016; Zarlenga et al., 1994; Zhu et al., 1998). The standard approach has been to amplify an appropriate taxonomic marker locus by PCR and clone and/or directly sequence it by Sanger (1st generation) sequencing. Different taxonomic markers can be used with their resolution depending on the of degree interspecies and intraspecies sequence variation in the taxonomic group(s) being examined. For example, the nuclear 18S and 28S rDNA coding gene markers are more conserved than the intervening ITS-1 and ITS-2 transcribed spacer regions and mtDNA markers, such as the cytochrome oxidase I (COI) and NADH-ubiquinone oxidoreductase chain 4 (ND4) genes being even less conserved (Dorris et al., 1999).

The choice of taxonomic marker also depends on other factors such as the target sequence length, the ease of sequence alignment and primer design and the availability of references for the species of interest. Detailed discussion of these issues for eukaryotic barcoding in general are available elsewhere (Beebe, 2018; Blaalid et al., 2013; Chan et al., 2021; Wang et al., 2015; Xia et al., 2012; Xu, 2016). Overall, the 18S rRNA gene has been the most common choice for nematode systematics. However, it has insufficient inter-species variation between closely related species in some nematode groups, including the order Strongylida which includes many of the important parasitic GIN of livestock and companion animals (Blaxter et al., 1998; Holterman et al., 2006). Consequently, the most commonly used marker for discriminating GIN species in domestic animal hosts has been the ITS-2 rRNA gene with mtDNA markers, typically COI and ND4, being generally used to assess within-species genetic diversity (Avramenko et al., 2015; Gasser et al., 2008).

4.7.2 Next-generation sequencing in GIN diagnostics

DNA barcoding using Sanger sequencing has been, and still is, valuable for the identification of individual specimens. However, the low scalability has limited its use for many diagnostic, surveillance or research applications. Nevertheless, the advent of next-generation massively parallel sequencing technologies now allows very large numbers of parasites to be synchronously sequenced at depth in large numbers of samples. In the case of domestic animal GINs, this allows the species and genetic composition of parasite communities in faecal samples to be accurately defined, providing a much wider range of diagnostic applications.

'Next generation' sequencing (NGS) technologies comprise several high-throughput sequencing approaches based on the concept of massively parallel sequencing. In essence these new technologies synchronously sequence very large numbers (many millions) of DNA molecules in parallel. This contrasts with 'first generation' sequencing methods, such as Sanger sequencing, in which a single DNA fragment is sequenced at a time. These 'next generation' sequencing methods are generally divided into two categories: 'Second generation', or massively parallel short-read sequencing, which is characterised by the amplification of short DNA templates, either on a solid phase flow cell or in an emulsion, followed by sequencing by synthesis (Heather and Chain, 2016). Although several different platforms have been developed, Illumina has become the dominant system in recent years. More recently, 'third generation' massively parallel sequencing has become available which is characterised by the sequencing of individual long strands of nucleic acid in real time. The main third generation sequencing platforms are Single Molecule Real Time (SMRT) (Pacific Biosciences) and nanopore sequencing (Oxford Nanopore Technologies) (Goto et al., 2019; Mohammadi and Bavi, 2021).

Next-generation sequencing technologies can potentially be used in a variety of ways for GIN parasite diagnostics. In theory, whole genome sequencing could be applied to DNA made from parasite communities extracted from faecal samples, or even DNA made directly from whole stool, in an approach equivalent to metagenomics used in microbiome studies. However, there are currently some major challenges for this approach in GIN diagnostics. Relative to bacterial species, nematodes have large and complex genomes (100–500 Mb in size) and there are still a limited number of drafts, and even fewer finished, reference whole genome sequences of GIN species from livestock and companion animal hosts (Coghlan et al., 2019).

Further, even if parasite stages in faeces can be efficiently lysed in DNA stool preparations, parasite DNA still constitutes a small proportion of the total genomic DNA extracted from stool. Consequently, to provide good representation and sufficient depth of coverage of the parasite community present, whole genome metagenomics requires huge sequencing depth, and so is still very costly. Furthermore, such data are currently challenging to analyse and interpret due to insufficient reference genome resources for the major parasite species of interest as well as the very high levels of sequence polymorphism (Coghlan et al., 2019; Gilleard and Redman, 2016). Because of this, the most practical application of next generation sequencing in GIN diagnostics is currently through deep sequencing of amplicons of specific targeted loci that have been generated by PCR from parasite populations harvested in faeces. Examples of loci of interest include rRNA or mtDNA taxonomic markers for species identification or loci carrying resistance mutations for anthelmintic resistance diagnostics.

To date, both Illumina short-read and SMRT long-read sequencing technologies have been used for diagnostic, surveillance and epidemiological research studies of domestic animal GIN. Although they are not yet used in commercial diagnostic laboratory settings, the rapid development of sequencing technologies offers huge potential for routine diagnostics. This is particularly the case for nanopore sequencing due to its potential to provide a combination of long-read sequence data, flexibility of sample size and low infrastructure costs. Although its application in parasite diagnostics has been limited to date by high sequencing error rates, this has been improved recently. The rapid development of sequencing technologies means this is a fast-changing field and likely to translate into routine diagnostics in veterinary medicine over the next few years as is beginning to occur in human medicine (Sheka et al., 2021).

The two main applications of next-generation deep amplicon sequencing in molecular diagnostics of GIN of domestic animals to date are ITS-2 rRNA gene metabarcoding for relative quantitation of species present in faecal samples, so-called nemabiome metabarcoding, and the detection and relative quantitation of single nucleotide polymorphism anthelmintic resistance mutations. We will deal with each of these in turn.

4.7.3 ITS-2 rRNA gene nemabiome metabarcoding methodologies

Nemabiome metabarcoding is essentially large-scale DNA barcoding using massively parallel sequencing technology to allow tens to hundreds of thousands of DNA molecules in a PCR amplicon to be sequenced simultaneously. In doing so, the targeted taxonomic marker is sequenced at depth from a large number of parasites in a sample, not only identifying the parasite species present but also providing information on their relative abundance.

ITS-2 rDNA metabarcoding was first described for GIN in domestic animals for cattle and the concept of the 'nemabiome' was introduced by analogy with 16S rDNA metabarcoding used in bacterial microbiome studies (Avramenko et al., 2015). The approach described by Avramenko et al. (2015) is a two-step PCR. The first PCR step amplifies the target ITS-2 rDNA and the second limited cycle PCR introduces indices and adapters required for Illumina sequencing (see Fig. 3 for details). The first round PCR amplification uses primers NC1 and NC2 that are complementary to the 5.8S and 28S sequences immediately adjacent to the ITS-2 rDNA target locus (Gasser et al., 1993). Primer site conservation eliminates the need to design and optimise species-specific primers for each target species of interest. The NC1 and NC2 primers are conserved across most Clade V nematodes, and so will amplify most of the important cattle, sheep and goat GIN. However, they are not as conserved across other nematode clades and so other first round PCR primers need to be considered depending on the taxonomic group(s) of interest. The second round PCR reaction introduces combinatorial indices (Fig. 3) allowing typically up to 384 samples to be pooled and sequenced in a single Miseq run depending on the sequence depth required for the particular application (Fig. 4). This, together with the large sequencing capacity of the Miseq platform, makes the approach extremely powerful and economical for large-scale studies. It also means that the method is extremely sensitive (Avramenko et al., 2015). However, in practice the true sensitivity is determined by a variety of factors including the number of parasites used to prepare the DNA sample and the quality of contamination control and quality assurance in the workflow. Protocol details are available at https://www.nemabiome.ca/analysis.html.

ITS-2 rDNA nemabiome metabarcoding has also recently been developed for sheep GIN using the Single Molecule Real Time (SMRT) (Pacific Biosciences) platform (Halvarsson and Höglund, 2021). There are advantages and disadvantages to the different next-generation sequencing platforms. The SMRT platform is not as widely available as the Illumina Miseq platform and cost per sample is higher due to the lower sequencing output, but it has the potential to provide greater resolution of species by sequencing longer taxonomic markers. Ultimately the choice at present may largely depend on the local equipment and expertise available.

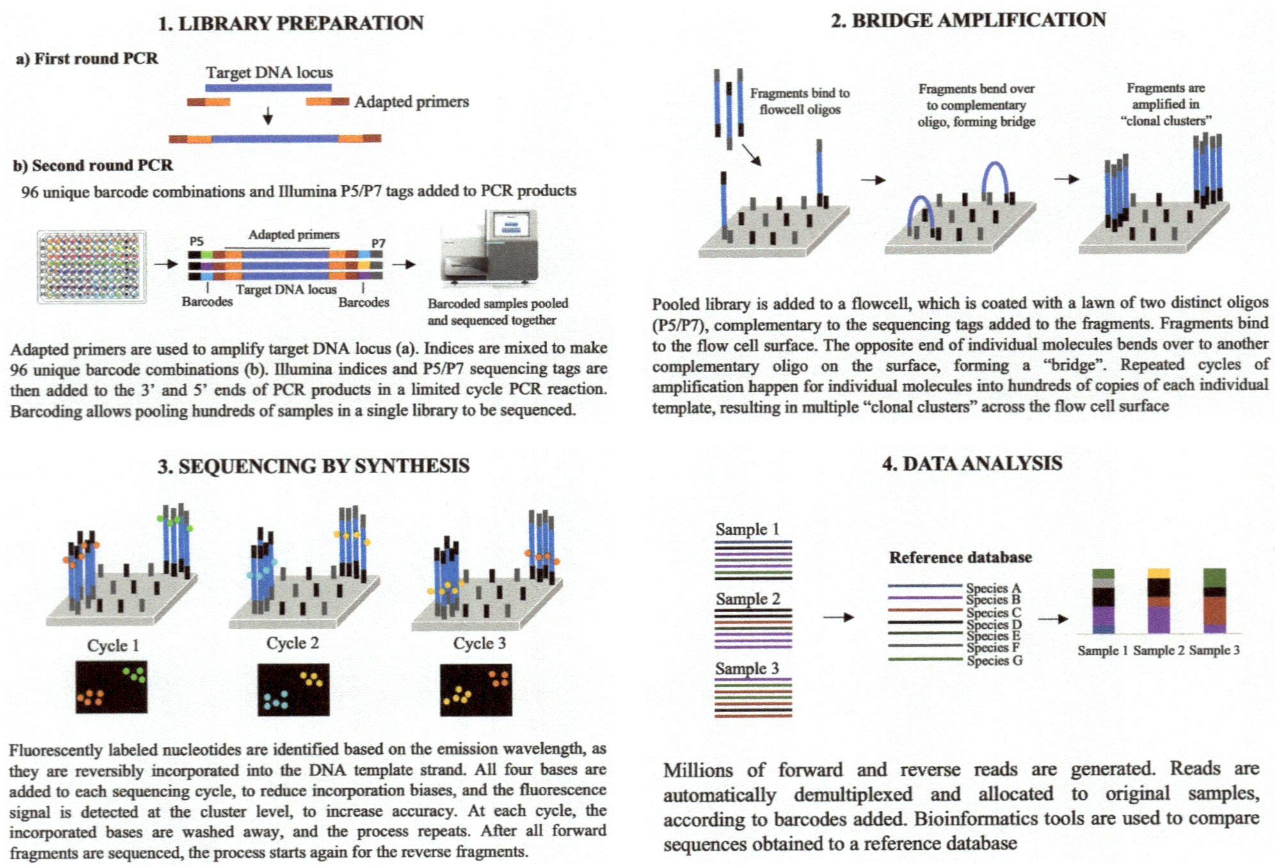

Fig. 3 Steps of nemabiome metabarcoding or deep amplicon sequencing using the Illumina short-read platform.

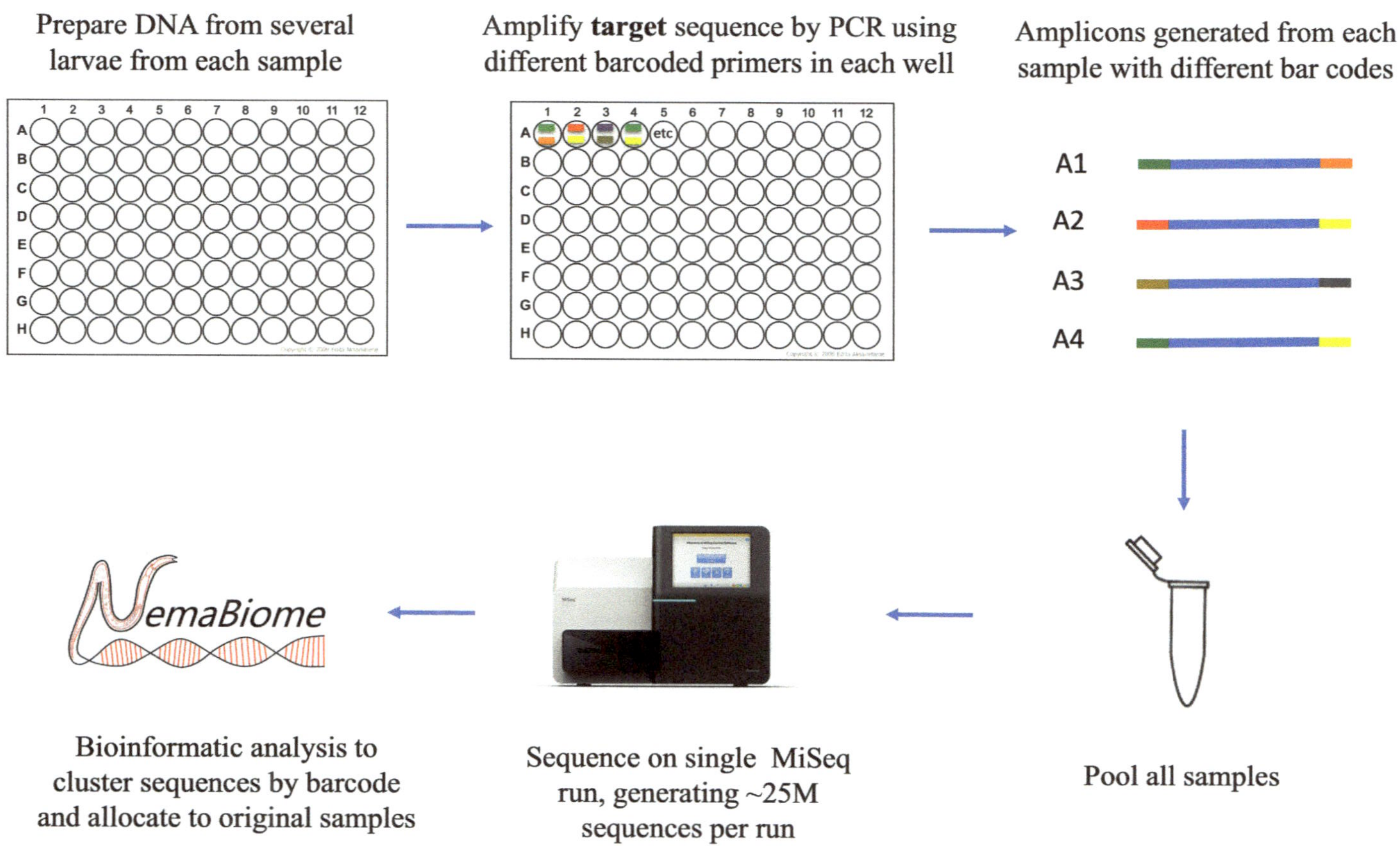

Fig. 4 Typical nemabiome metabarcoding or deep amplicon sequencing workflow.

The large sequencing capacity of NGS platforms, which in the case of the Miseq is up to 25 million paired-end reads per run, means it is well suited for large scale studies, in situations where sets of samples can be batched, but uneconomic for small numbers of samples. Ongoing developments in sequencing technology and platforms, such as nanopore sequencing using the MINION and Flongle devices (Avershina et al., 2022), are likely to both improve flexibility and reduce costs in the future.

4.7.4 Nemabiome metabarcoding data analysis

Methods for the analysis of the large amount of sequence data generated by short read Illumina ITS-2 rDNA nemabiome metabarcoding are continuously evolving and details, which are beyond the scope of this review, are available at https://www.nemabiome.ca/analysis.html. The original ITS-2 rDNA nemabiome metabarcoding method used a Mothur-based bioinformatic pipeline (Schloss et al., 2009) and this is still a valuable approach for cattle and sheep diagnostics. More recently, dada2-based pipelines have been used to generate Amplified Sequence Variants (ASVs) which can potentially provide greater resolution, particularly for closely related species and also better capture the within-species diversity (Callahan et al., 2015, 2017). The validity of species identification using metabarcoding depends on a number of factors, including the appropriateness of the chosen taxonomic marker, the sequence quality, the sequence filtering and the method used for taxonomic assignment of sequences, of which a number have been used including Mothur, Assign Taxonomy, IDTaxa and Blast (Avramenko et al., 2015; Beaumelle et al., 2021). In the case of ITS-2 rDNA nemabiome metabarcoding using SMRT sequencing (Pacific Biosciences), a different analysis approach and pipeline has been used to cluster ITS-2 sequences into OTUs with an analysis framework, SCATA, specifically designed for eukaryotes (Halvarsson and Höglund, 2021).

Another important consideration is the choice and quality of the reference sequence database used. The public databases such as GenBank are far from perfect and contain many partial ITS-2 sequences, submissions with inaccurate species labels and a huge variance in the number of submissions for different species, all of which can lead to species misassignment. Consequently, curated databases are needed, with the choice depending on the details of the application. For example, a manually curated ITS-2 rDNA database restricted to relevant, reliably identified, full-length ITS-2 rDNA reference sequences has been used for domestic ruminant diagnostics (Avramenko et al., 2015). However, this restricted database is not suitable if either the target GIN species are not known, such as in geographical regions with little information on parasite fauna, or in many wildlife host species. A more comprehensive database is available for such situations that currently includes 11,297 non-redundant full-length ITS-2 rDNA sequences from 1637 nematode species and which is automatically updated from GenBank several times each year https://www.nemabiome.ca/its2-database.html (Workentine et al., 2020). There is an ongoing need for database improvement, including more robustly validated reference sequences, additional nematode species and inclusion of sequences from a wider variety of geographical regions.

4.7.5 Determination of relative species abundance using nemabiome metabarcoding

Nemabiome metabarcoding provides information on the relative abundance of nematode species by sequencing at depth the targeted taxonomic marker in the parasite population. Typically, 10,000 of sequences are generated from each sample and the number of sequences assigning to each species reflects their relative abundance in the sample. However, there are a number of important factors to consider.

Firstly, the number, or at least the minimum number, of parasites used to prepare the DNA needs to be known. Amplicons can be generated and sequenced from a single egg or larvae but, clearly, preparing DNA from a very small number of eggs or larvae will not provide meaningful information on relative abundance of species present in a sample or host. It is not possible to provide universal guidelines on the minimum number of parasites required as it will vary depending on the complexity of the parasite population and the quantitative accuracy required for the particular diagnostic application. For sheep and cattle, the minimum number of larvae used in published studies has varied from 100 to 1,000 (Avramenko et al., 2017; Evans et al., 2021; Queiroz et al., 2020; Redman et al., 2019).

Secondly, the relative number of sequences mapping to a particular species does not directly measure the relative number of organisms and there are many potential sources of bias. As with any PCR-based method, there are likely differences in the efficiency of DNA lysis or in PCR amplification efficiency between species, even for conserved primers. In addition, the amount of DNA per individual can potentially vary between species, even of the same developmental stage, due to differing cell or nuclei number or the copy number of the target locus. In the case of ITS-2 rDNA, copy numbers have been shown to vary from 50 to 200 copies for different nematode species (Bik et al., 2013).

Another source of bias can be the stage of development of different species in a sample. Different species develop at different rates and so can potentially have different cell numbers/DNA content, depending on the age and storage conditions of a faecal sample when the DNA is prepared. It is difficult, if not impossible, to control for all these potential confounders, which equally apply to other molecular diagnostic methods, and so empirical testing and careful methodological standardization is required to maximise the accuracy of relative abundance determination. For sheep and cattle GIN, experiments with mock larval communities of known GIN species composition have shown that ITS-2 rDNA nemabiome metabarcoding provides reasonably accurate estimates of relative species abundance in spite of all the potential confounding factors (Avramenko et al., 2015; Redman et al., 2019). In addition, for these two host species, correction factors have been empirically determined, using data from these mock community experiments, to improve the accuracy of species relative abundance determination (Avramenko et al., 2015; Redman et al., 2019).

Different parasite stages present in faeces—eggs, L1 or L3 larvae can be specifically targeted for nemabiome metabarcoding and the best choice will vary depending on the application. The original ITS-2 rDNA nemabiome metabarcoding method was applied to L3 from bovine coprocultures, partly to allow method validation more easily and partly because of the ease of harvesting large numbers of L3; setting up large coprocultures is much less labour intensive than harvesting of large numbers of eggs by flotation when faecal egg counts are low, as is often the case in cattle (Avramenko et al., 2015). Nemabiome metabarcoding has subsequently been applied to eggs, harvested by flotation, or L1s following controlled hatching of harvested eggs (Borkowski et al., 2020; Francis and Šlapeta, 2022; Queiroz et al., 2020; Redman et al., 2019). The correlation between the data generated from eggs, L1 and L3 has been found to be good overall (Francis and Šlapeta, 2022; Redman et al., 2019) although differences can occur depending on the coproculture conditions (Borkowski et al., 2020). Most recently, nemabiome metabarcoding has been applied directly to DNA made from stool (Francis and Šlapeta, 2022). One important area for further development is improvement of methods for faecal sample preparation and/or harvesting and concentrating of parasites from faeces to improve the speed, efficiency, and reliability of these steps in the process.

4.7.6 Application of nemabiome metabarcoding in veterinary diagnostics

ITS-2 rDNA nemabiome metabarcoding has now been developed and applied for relative species quantitation of GIN for a number of domestic livestock host species, including cattle, sheep, horses, and bison (Avramenko et al., 2017, 2018; Mitchell et al., 2019; Poissant et al., 2021; Redman et al., 2019). It has also been used to determine hookworm species identity in dogs although it has not yet been as widely applied in companion animals (Jimenez Castro et al., 2019, 2021). Its use in wild animal host species is beyond the scope of this review but details are available elsewhere (Aivelo and Medlar, 2017; Barone et al., 2020; Beaumelle et al., 2021). There are a variety of diagnostic applications and some of the main ones to date are discussed below and the advantages and disadvantages of the approach are summarised in Box 2.

ITS-2 rDNA nemabiome metabarcoding is a powerful tool for large-scale surveillance and epidemiological studies because prevalence and relative infection intensity data can be generated for multiple parasite species from hundreds of animals and/or farms in a single sequencing run. For example, the relative abundance of the 8 most common ovine GIN

BOX 2 Advantages and Disadvantages of nemabiome metabarcoding in domestic animal GIN diagnostics.

Advantages	Disadvantages
Accurate identification of GIN to species level	Currently requires batching of large numbers of samples to make economic
Doesn't require assay optimization for each individual target species	Set up costs are relatively high
Can identify unexpected species present in samples	Bioinformatic expertise required
Can be standardised between labs	Strict workflows and analysis protocols to control contamination and bar code hopping
Less specialised expertise needed	Current use has been to research applications due to disadvantages listed above
More objective than microscopy-based methods	

was determined using a single PCR for each sample from 93 groups of ewes and 61 groups of lambs derived from 99 UK sheep farms on a single Illumina Miseq run (Redman et al., 2019). Similar surveys have been undertaken in sheep in other regions as well as in beef cattle, dairy cattle and bison (Avramenko et al., 2017, 2018; Costa-Junior et al., 2021; Evans et al., 2021; Scott et al., 2019). It is also a powerful tool for detailed longitudinal monitoring, epidemiological studies and assessing control programmes. For example, it was used to determine the relative GIN species abundance in faecal samples from groups of ewes and lambs at 3–4 week intervals between spring and autumn over a period of 4 years on a commercial farm in south-eastern Scotland (Costa-Junior et al., 2021; Evans et al., 2021). It has also been applied to environmental samples to investigate the survival of infective larvae of different cattle GIN species over the winter as well as their rate of accumulation on pastures during the grazing season (Wang et al., 2020, 2021).

Another application has been in anthelmintic efficacy testing and resistance diagnostics (Avramenko et al., 2017; Costa-Junior et al., 2021; Halvarsson and Höglund, 2021; Queiroz et al., 2020). A major limitation of FECRT tests in livestock is the lack of GIN species information that is provided by faecal strongyle egg counts, which reduces the sensitivity of the test and provides challenges for interpretation. An example addressing these limitations was a study which integrated the FECRT and ITS-2 rDNA nemabiome metabarcoding to reveal that ivermectin and fenbendazole resistance was common in *H. contortus* but much less common in *T. circumcincta* and *T. colubriformis* in western Canadian sheep flocks and also suggested early emergence of levamisole resistance in *T. circumcincta* (Queiroz et al., 2020). The study also revealed that the poor efficacy detected by the FECRT to closantel on a number of farms was due to its narrow spectrum of activity rather than to anthelmintic resistance. There is a need to improve practical workflows to make such approaches more suitable for routine diagnostics in clinical practice. An interesting recent technical development is the application to eggs harvested directly from FECPAK chambers following egg counting (Francis and Šlapeta, 2022). This, and other similar approaches, could open the way to more routine use in herd health programmes.

4.7.7 Deep amplicon sequencing to detect and determine the frequency of anthelmintic resistance associated SNPs

The ability to detect and quantify drug resistance mutations in parasite populations has the potential to provide much more sensitive, accurate and scalable diagnostic tests of anthelmintic resistance than the current *in vivo* and *in vitro* tests (Kotze et al., 2020). At present, the benzimidazoles are the only anthelmintics for which the major causal mutations are known with confidence, which is the case for multiple ruminant GIN species. An Illumina short-read deep amplicon sequencing assay has been developed to determine the frequency of benzimidazole resistance mutations at codons 167, 198 and 200 of the isotype-1 β-tubulin gene of the major ovine GIN (Avramenko et al., 2019).

The basic methodology is similar to ITS-2 rDNA metabarcoding but instead, targets the isotype-1 β-tubulin gene encoding the benzimidazole drug target. An assay was developed based on deep sequencing of amplicons generated from a multiplex PCR, targeting the relevant section of the isotype-1 β-tubulin gene from multiple bovine GIN species including *H. contortus*, *T. circumcincta*, *T. colubriformis*, *T. axei*, *T. vitrinus*, and *Cooperia curticei* for deep sequencing. This assay allowed the simultaneous screening for benzimidazole resistance mutations at all three codons for the six major ovine GIN parasite species from 95 groups of ewes and 69 groups of lambs from flocks across the United Kingdom in a single MiSeq sequencing run (Avramenko et al., 2019). A similar approach was used to target *T. circumcincta* and used to monitor benzimidazole resistance mutations over a 4-year period on a commercial sheep farm (Evans et al., 2021; Sargison et al., 2019a). The approach has also been used for benzimidazole resistance surveillance in cattle and bison GIN (Avramenko et al., 2020; Jimenez Castro et al., 2021) and recently in dogs to survey greyhounds across the United States for benzimidazole resistance in *Ancylostoma caninum* (Jimenez Castro et al., 2021).

The major limiting factor at present for the application of these approaches to other anthelmintic drug classes and parasite species is our incomplete understanding of the mutations underlying resistance. However, the recent progress made for ruminant GIN for other drug classes such as levamisole and macrocyclic lactones may allow more comprehensive resistance mutations assays to be developed in the foreseeable future, as has been discussed in a recent review (Kotze et al., 2020).

5. Decision-making based on diagnosis

Diagnosis of parasite infection provides valuable evidence for effective worm control but the application of diagnostic tools in practice depends on multiple factors including ease-of-use, cost and the value of information. It is crucial for the advisers and animal owners to understand the results correctly and to incorporate them into a decision-making process. Relying on a single test result can be misleading and, in most cases, multiple factors need to be considered before diagnostic test results can be interpreted in terms of control decisions. Guidelines on how to apply diagnostics and how to interpret test results are increasingly available for the different domestic species.

The decision-making process could be considered most straightforward in companion animals. Given the close relationships with human and the importance of several zoonotic species, the general advice and desire from the owners is to keep them parasite free. Aiming to protect both the health of the pets and the public, ESCCAP (European Scientific Counsel Companion Animal Parasites) recommends pet-specific worm control schemes based on individual assessment of risk factors. For example, the frequency of annual faecal examination depends on the pet's lifestyle and exposure risks and is categorised into four different groups. The guideline has been used to evaluate worm control status in several countries such as Germany (Strube et al., 2019) and France (Roussel et al., 2019). Another important resource in the United States is CAPC (Companion Animal Parasite Council). A useful feature on this website is the monthly parasite prevalence map which is developed using diagnostic data from the United States and Canada (available at: https://capcvet.org/maps/#/). Although only representing less than 30% of the parasite diagnostic activity in these geographic regions, the data provide timely information for the diagnosis and prevalence of parasite in each province.

Diagnosis-driven decision-making in the livestock industry is often more complicated than companion animals because rather than treating when an infection is diagnosed, intervention is only recommended when certain infection thresholds are exceeded and should take into account the impact of infection on productivity (Charlier et al., 2014) and farm economics (van der Voort et al., 2013). Moreover, control is compounded by the problem of AR (Charlier et al., 2022). Information about evidence-based parasite control is often available on regional websites and labs. The industry-led multi-stakeholder initiatives SCOPS (sustainable control of parasites in sheep), COWS (control of worms sustainable) in the United Kingdom (Taylor, 2012) and the ACSRPC (American Consortium for Small Ruminant Parasite Control) in the United States may serve as good examples. FEC monitoring plays an important role in the recommendations made by these initiatives. Studies have shown that farms implementing SCOPS guidelines (e.g. effective quarantine drenching, selective treatment of lambs, etc.) used less anthelmintic treatments than traditionally managed farms, without loss of animal performance or increased worm burden (Learmount et al., 2016; Williams et al., 2021). However, a wide range of socio-psychological, economic and practical constraints exert uncertainties on the uptake of such practice by farmers. Future recommendations should focus on transparent benefits and practical applications to maintain long-term positive behavioural change (Jack et al., 2022).

Although diagnostics are traditionally being used to inform anthelmintic treatment decisions, given the continuing spread of AR, diagnostics will increasingly underpin the use of other, complementary control options, including breeding, grazing management, plant or fungi-based control and vaccines (Charlier et al., 2022) These complementary control options are also referred to as the 'Basket of Options', aiming to provide practical and affordable parasite interventions to farmers and reducing the need to rely on anthelmintics for strategic nematode control (Krecek and Waller, 2006). The COST Action project COMBAR (https://www.combar-ca.eu) further developed this concept into a catalogue, setting out the various options that can be applied based on different farm situations. Diagnostics guide the targeted use of all the options in the basket. Indicators (e.g. FEC, bulk tank antibodies and pepsinogen) and control options are described from a practical angle and supported by case studies in the field to help uptake by the readers.

Another tool, building on diagnostic test results to understand the farm-level production and economic impact, is ParaCalc®. It is a spreadsheet model to estimate the costs of parasitic infections or treatment strategies on dairy farms based on herd-specific diagnostic test results (Charlier et al., 2012). It can be expected that the digital revolution will spur the development of completely new decision support systems, for instance, building on deep learning networks (Tekin et al., 2021), species identification via sequencing tools (Vercruysse et al., 2018), and the correlations between animal (grazing) behaviour and helminth infection that are beginning to be unravelled (Högberg et al., 2021).

6. Conclusions and way forward

This review summarised recent advances in the diagnosis of GIN in livestock and companion animals. In the last decades, diagnostic tools and techniques used in veterinary parasitology have been harmonised and have evolved rapidly through exploitation of machine learning and artificial intelligence for automated parasite egg counting as well as biomarker identification of nematodes using innovative molecular and proteomic methods. Furthermore, efforts have been made towards a holistic approach that considers the fundamental role of diagnosis to guide treatment strategies in order to avoid the threat of drug resistance. We call for a broad and synergistic approach to surveillance and control of parasitic infections of animals through combination of a set of advanced and standardised diagnostic methods. The 2030 veterinary toolbox should be equipped with advanced diagnostic methods to tackle parasitic infections of farm and companion animals. Research pipelines for improved diagnostics should be expanded and transferred to the key stakeholders along with efforts for developing vaccines and new therapeutics as well as complementary control approaches.

Acknowledgements

This article is based in part upon work from COST Action COMBAR CA16230, supported by COST (European Cooperation in Science and Technology). It is also based upon work conducted by the STAR-IDAZ IRC Scientific sub-Committee "Diagnostic test roadmap" developed by the Livestock Helminth Research Alliance (LiHRA; June 2019) with major contributions of John Gilleard, Georg von Samson Himmelstjerna, Diana Williams, Laura Rinaldi, Edwin Claerebout, Peter Geldhof and Jozef Vercruysse.

References

Aboshady, H.M., Stear, M.J., Johansson, A., Jonas, E., Bambou, J.C., 2020. Immunoglobulins as biomarkers for gastrointestinal nematodes resistance in small ruminants: A systematic review. Sci. Rep. 10 (1), 1–14.

Acosta Soto, L., Santísima-Trinidad, A.B., Bornay-Llinares, F.J., Martín González, M., Pascual Valero, J.A., Ros Muñoz, M., 2017. Quantitative PCR and digital PCR for detection of *Ascaris lumbricoides* eggs in reclaimed water. Biomed. Res. Int. 2017 (7515409).

Ademola, I.O., Krucken, J., Ramunke, S., Demeler, J., von Samson-Himmelstjerna, G., 2015. Absence of detectable benzimidazole-resistance associated alleles in *Haemonchus placei* in cattle in Nigeria revealed by pyrosequencing of beta-tubulin isotype 1. Parasitol. Res. 114 (5), 1997–2001.

Adolph, C., Barnett, S., Beall, M., Drake, J., Elsemore, D., Thomas, J., Little, S., 2017. Diagnostic strategies to reveal covert infections with intestinal helminths in dogs. Vet. Parasitol. 247, 108–112.

Aivelo, T., Medlar, A., 2017. Opportunities and challenges in metabarcoding approaches for helminth community identification in wild mammals. Parasitology 145, 608–621.

Aliabadi, J., Rakhshandehroo, E., Yektaseresht, A., 2021. Development and evaluation of an indirect ELISA for detection of *Teladorsagia circumcincta* infection in sheep. BMC Vet. Res. 17 (1), 1–9.

Amoah, I.D., Singh, G., Troell, K., Reddy, P., Stenström, T.A., Bux, F., 2020. Comparative assessment of DNA extraction procedures for *ascaris* spp. eggs. J. Helminthol. 94, e78.

Andersen, U.V., Howe, D.K., Dangoudoubiyam, S., Toft, N., Reinemeyer, C.R., Lyons, E.T., Olsen, S.N., Monrad, J., Nejsum, P., Nielsen, M.K., 2013a. SvSXP: A *Strongylus vulgaris* antigen with potential for prepatent diagnosis. Parasit. Vectors 6 (1), 1–13.

Andersen, U.V., Howe, D.K., Olsen, S.N., Nielsen, M.K., 2013b. Recent advances in diagnosing pathogenic equine gastrointestinal helminths: the challenge of prepatent detection. Vet. Parasitol. 192 (1–3), 1–9.

Andreasen, A., Petersen, H.H., Kringel, H., Iburg, T.M., Skovgaard, K., Dawson, H., Urban, J.F., Thamsborg, S.M., 2015. Immune and inflammatory responses in pigs infected with *Trichuris suis* and *Oesophagostomum dentatum*. Vet. Parasitol. 207 (3–4), 249–258.

Antinori, S., Ridolfo, A.L., Grande, R., Galimberti, L., Casalini, G., Giacomelli, A., Milazzo, L., 2021. Loop-mediated isothermal amplification (lamp) assay for the diagnosis of imported malaria: A narrative review. Infez. Med. 29, 355–365.

Avershina, E., Frye, S.A., Ali, J., Taxt, A.M., Ahmad, R., 2022. Ultrafast and cost-effective pathogen identification and resistance gene detection in a clinical setting using nanopore Flongle sequencing. Front. Microbiol. 13.

Avila, H.G., Risso, M.G., Cabrera, M., Ruybal, P., Repetto, S.A., Butti, M.J., Trangoni, M.D., Santillán, G., Pérez, V.M., Periago, M.V., 2021a. Development of a new LAMP assay for the detection of *Ancylostoma caninum* DNA (Copro-LAMPAc) in dog fecal samples. Front. Vet. Sci. 8, 1–8.

Avila, H.G., Risso, M.G., Ruybal, P., Repetto, S.A., Butti, M.J., Trangoni, M.D., Grune Löffler, S., Pérez, V.M., Periago, M.V., 2021b. Development of a low-cost copro-LAMP assay for simultaneous copro-detection of *Toxocara canis* and *Toxocara cati*. Parasitology 148, 819–826.

Avramenko, R.W., Redman, E.M., Lewis, R., Yazwinski, T.A., Wasmuth, J.D., Gilleard, J.S., 2015. Exploring the gastrointestinal "Nemabiome": deep amplicon sequencing to quantify the species composition of parasitic nematode communities. PLoS One 10.

Avramenko, R.W., Redman, E.M., Lewis, R., Bichuette, M.A., Palmeira, B.M., Yazwinski, T.A., Gilleard, J.S., 2017. The use of nemabiome metabarcoding to explore gastro-intestinal nematode species diversity and anthelmintic treatment effectiveness in beef calves. Int. J. Parasitol. 47, 893–902.

Avramenko, R.W., Bras, A., Redman, E.M., Woodbury, M.R., Wagner, B., Shury, T., Liccioli, S., Windeyer, M.C., Gilleard, J.S., 2018. High species diversity of trichostrongyle parasite communities within and between Western Canadian commercial and conservation bison herds revealed by nemabiome metabarcoding. Parasit. Vectors 11, 299.

Avramenko, R.W., Redman, E.M., Melville, L., Bartley, Y., Wit, J., Queiroz, C., Bartley, D.J., Gilleard, J.S., 2019. Deep amplicon sequencing as a powerful new tool to screen for sequence polymorphisms associated with anthelmintic resistance in parasitic nematode populations. Int. J. Parasitol. 49, 13–26.

Avramenko, R.W., Redman, E.M., Windeyer, C., Gilleard, J.S., 2020. Assessing anthelmintic resistance risk in the post-genomic era: a proof-of-concept study assessing the potential for widespread benzimidazole-resistant gastrointestinal nematodes in north American cattle and bison. Parasitology 147, 897–906.

Ayana, M., Vlaminck, J., Cools, P., Ame, S., Albonico, M., Dana, D., Keiser, J., Manly, H., Matoso, L.F., Mekonnen, Z., Montresor, A., Correa-Oliveira, R., Rinaldi, L., Sayasone, S., Sowersby, S.J., Tesfaye, L., Vercruysse, J., Mirams, G., Levecke, B., 2018. Modification and optimization of the $FECPAK^{G2}$ protocol for the detection and quantification of soil-transmitted helminth eggs in human stool. PLoS Negl. Trop. Dis. 12 (10), e0006655.

Ayana, M., Cools, P., Mekonnen, Z., Biruksew, A., Dana, D., Rashwan, N., Prichard, R., Vlaminck, J., Verweij, J.J., Levecke, B., 2019. Comparison of four DNA extraction and three preservation protocols for the molecular detection and quantification of soil-transmitted helminths in stool. PLoS Negl. Trop. Dis. 13, e0007778.

Azimian, H., Shokrani, H., Fallahi, S., 2021. Molecular evaluation of *Toxocara* species in stray cats using loop-mediated isothermal amplification (lamp) technique as a rapid, sensitive and simple screening assay. Vet. Med. Sci. 7, 647–653.

Azzopardi, K.I., Hardy, M., Baker, C., Bonnici, R., Llewellyn, S., McCarthy, J.S., Traub, R.J., Steer, A.C., 2021. Detection of six soil-transmitted helminths in human stool by qPCR - a systematic workflow. PLoS One 16, e0258039.

Balinsky, D.L., Paras, K.L., Hanna, R., Elsemore, D.A., Verocai, G.G., 2019. Parasite survey on a captive wolf population using classical techniques and ELISA coproantigen detection, USA. Vet. Parasitol.: Reg. Stud. Rep. 16, 100285.

Ballweber, L.R., Beugnet, F., Marchiondo, A.A., Payne, P.A., 2014. American Association of Veterinary Parasitologists' review of veterinary fecal flotation methods and factors influencing their accuracy and use- -is there really one best technique? Vet. Parasitol. 204 (1–2), 73–80.

Baltrušis, P., Halvarsson, P., Höglund, J., 2018. Exploring benzimidazole resistance in *Haemonchus contortus* by next generation sequencing and droplet digital PCR. *International journal for parasitology*. Drug Resist. 8, 411–419.

Baltrušis, P., Halvarsson, P., Höglund, J., 2019. Molecular detection of two major gastrointestinal parasite genera in cattle using a novel droplet digital PCR approach. Parasitol. Res. 118, 2901–2907.

Baltrušis, P., Halvarsson, P., Höglund, J., 2020. Utilization of droplet digital PCR to survey resistance associated polymorphisms in the β tubulin gene of *Haemonchus contortus* in sheep flocks in Sweden. Vet. Parasitol. 288, 109278.

Barone, C.D., Wit, J., Hoberg, E.P., Gilleard, J.S., Zarlenga, D.S., 2020. Wild ruminants as reservoirs of domestic livestock gastrointestinal nematodes. Vet. Parasitol. 279, 109041.

Barrere, V., Falzon, L.C., Shakya, K.P., Menzies, P.I., Peregrine, A.S., Prichard, R.K., 2013. Assessment of benzimidazole resistance in *Haemonchus contortus* in sheep flocks in Ontario, Canada: comparison of detection methods for drug resistance. Vet. Parasitol. 198, 159–165.

Basripuzi, N.H., Salisi, M.S., Isa, N., Busin, V., Cairns, C., Jenvey, C., Stear, M.J., 2018. Boer goats appear to lack a functional IgA and eosinophil response against natural nematode infection. Vet. Parasitol. 264, 18–25.

Basuni, M., Muhi, J., Othman, N., Verweij, J.J., Ahmad, M., Miswan, N., Rahumatullah, A., Aziz, F.A., Zainudin, N.S., Noordin, R., 2011. A pentaplex real-time polymerase chain reaction assay for detection of four species of soil-transmitted helminths. Am. J. Trop. Med. Hyg. 84, 338–343.

Basuni, M., Mohamed, Z., Ahmad, M., Zakaria, N.Z., Noordin, R., 2012. Detection of selected intestinal helminths and protozoa at hospital Universiti Sains Malaysia using multiplex realtime PCR. Trop. Biomed. 29, 434–442.

Baum, L., Ng, A., Leung, W.K., 2005. Developing the use of mismatch binding proteins for discovering rare somatic mutations. Mol. Cell. Probes 19, 163–168.

Beaumelle, C., Redman, E.M., de Rijke, J., Wit, J., Benabed, S., Debias, F., Duhayer, J., Pardonnet, S., Poirel, M.-T., Capron, G., Chabot, S., Rey, B., Yannic, G., Gilleard, J.S., Bourgoin, G., 2021. Metabarcoding in two isolated populations of wild roe deer (*Capreolus capreolus*) reveals variation in gastrointestinal nematode community composition between regions and among age classes. Parasit. Vectors 14, 594.

Beebe, N.W., 2018. DNA barcoding mosquitoes: advice for potential prospectors. Parasitology 145, 622–633.

Beims, R.F., Simonato, C.L., Wiggers, V.R., 2019. Technology readiness level assessment of pyrolysis of trygliceride biomass to fuels and chemicals. Renew. Sustain. Energy Rev. 112, 521–529.

Bellaw, J.L., Nielsen, M.K., 2020. Meta-analysis of cyathostomin species-specific prevalence and relative abundance in domestic horses from 1975-2020: emphasis on geographical region and specimen collection method. Parasit. Vectors 13 (1), 509.

Bik, H.M., Fournier, D., Sung, W., Bergeron, R.D., Thomas, W.K., 2013. Intra-genomic variation in the ribosomal repeats of nematodes. PLoS One 8, e78230.

Blaalid, R., Kumar, S., Nilsson, R.H., Abarenkov, K., Kirk, P.M., Kauserud, H., 2013. ITS1 versus ITS2 as DNA metabarcodes for fungi. Mol. Ecol. Resour. 13 (2), 218–224.

Blaxter, M.L., De Ley, P., Garey, J.R., Liu, L.X., Scheldeman, P., Vierstraete, A., Vanfleteren, J.R., Mackey, L.Y., Dorris, M., Frisse, L.M., Vida, J.T., Thomas, W.K., 1998. A molecular evolutionary framework for the phylum Nematoda. Nature 392, 71–75.

Boelow, H., Krücken, J., Thomas, E., Mirams, G., von Samson-Himmelstjerna, G., 2022. Comparison of FECPAK^{G2}, a modified mini-FLOTAC technique and combined sedimentation and flotation for the coproscopic examination of helminth eggs in horses. Parasit. Vectors 15 (1), 166.

Bøgh, H.O., Eriksen, L., Lawson, L.G., Lind, P., 1994. Evaluation of an enzyme-linked immunosorbent assay and a histamine release test system for the detection of pigs naturally infected with *ascaris suum*. Prev. Vet. Med. 21 (3), 201–214.

Borba, V.H., Martin, C., Machado-Silva, J.R., Xavier, S., de Mello, F.L., Iñiguez, A.M., 2021. Machine learning approach to support taxonomic species discrimination based on helminth collections data. Parasit. Vectors 14 (1), 230.

Borkowski, E.A., Redman, E.M., Chant, R., Avula, J., Menzies, P.I., Karrow, N.A., Lillie, B.N., Sears, W., Gilleard, J.S., Peregrine, A.S., 2020. Comparison of ITS-2 rDNA nemabiome sequencing with morphological identification to quantify gastrointestinal nematode community species composition in small ruminant feces. Vet. Parasitol. 282, 109104.

Bott, N.J., Campbell, B.E., Beveridge, I., Chilton, N.B., Rees, D., Hunt, P.W., Gasser, R.B., 2009. A combined microscopic-molecular method for the diagnosis of strongylid infections in sheep. Int. J. Parasitol. 39, 1277–1287.

Brasil, B.S.A.F., Nunes, R.L., Bastianetto, E., Drummond, M.G., Carvalho, D.C., Leite, R.C., Molento, M.B., Oliveira, D.A.A., 2012. Genetic diversity patterns of *Haemonchus placei* and *Haemonchus contortus* populations isolated from domestic ruminants in Brazil. Int. J. Parasitol. 42, 469–479.

Bredtmann, C.M., Krücken, J., Murugaiyan, J., Balard, A., Hofer, H., Kuzmina, T.A., von Samson-Himmelstjerna, G., 2019. Concurrent proteomic fingerprinting and molecular analysis of cyathostomins. Proteomics 19, e1800290.

Bungiro, R.D., Cappello, M., 2005. Detection of excretory/secretory coproantigens in experimental hookworm infection. Am. J. Trop. Med. Hyg. 73, 915–920.

Burk, S.V., Dangoudoubiyam, S., Brewster-Barnes, T., Bryant, U.K., Howe, D.K., Carter, C.N., Vanzant, E.S., Harmon, R.J., Kazacos, K.R., Rossano, M.G., 2014. *In vitro* culture of *Parascaris equorum* larvae and initial investigation of parasite excretory-secretory products. Parasitol. Res. 113 (11), 4217–4224.

Burk, S.V., Dangoudoubiyam, S., Brewster-Barnes, T., Howe, D.K., Carter, C.N., Bryant, U.K., Rossano, M.G., 2016. Equine antibody response to larval *Parascaris equorum* excretory-secretory products. Vet. Parasitol. 226, 83–87.

Cain, J.L., Slusarewicz, P., Rutledge, M.H., McVey, M.R., Wielgus, K.M., Zynda, H.M., Wehling, L.M., Scare, J.A., Steuer, A.E., Nielsen, M.K., 2020. Diagnostic performance of McMaster, Wisconsin, and automated egg counting techniques for enumeration of equine strongyle eggs in fecal samples. Vet. Parasitol. 284, 109199.

Cain, J.L., Peters, K.T., Suri, P., Roher, A., Rutledge, M.H., Nielsen, M.K., 2021. The effect of analyst training on fecal egg counting variability. Parasitol. Res. 120 (4), 1363–1370.

Callahan, B.J., McMurdie, P.J., Rosen, M.J., Han, A.W., Johnson, A.J., Holmes, S.P., 2015. DADA2: high resolution sample inference from amplicon data. Nat. Methods 13 (7), 581–583.

Callahan, B.J., McMurdie, P.J., Holmes, S.P., 2017. Exact sequence variants should replace operational taxonomic units in marker-gene data analysis. ISME J. 11, 2639–2643.

Campbell, B.E., Nisbet, A.J., Mulvenna, J., Loukas, A., Gasser, R.B., 2008. Molecular and phylogenetic characterization of cytochromes c from *Haemonchus contortus* and *Trichostrongylus vitrinus* (Nematoda: Trichostrongylida). Gene 424, 121–129.

Chan, A.H.E., Chaisiri, K., Saralamba, S., Morand, S., Thaenkham, U., 2021. Assessing the suitability of mitochondrial and nuclear DNA genetic markers for molecular systematics and species identification of helminths. Parasit. Vectors 14, 233.

Charlier, J., Claerebout, E., Duchateau, L., Vercruysse, J., 2005. A survey to determine relationships between bulk tank milk antibodies against *Ostertagia ostertagi* and milk production parameters. Vet. Parasitol. 129 (1–2), 67–75.

Charlier, J., Duchateau, L., Claerebout, E., Vercruysse, J., 2007. Predicting milk-production responses after an autumn treatment of pastured dairy herds with eprinomectin. Vet. Parasitol. 143 (3–4), 322–328.

Charlier, J., De Cat, A., Forbes, A., Vercruysse, J., 2009. Measurement of antibodies to gastrointestinal nematodes and liver fluke in meat juice of beef cattle and associations with carcass parameters. Vet. Parasitol. 166 (3–4), 235–240.

Charlier, J., Vercruysse, J., Smith, J., Vanderstichel, R., Stryhn, H., Claerebout, E., Dohoo, I., 2010. Evaluation of anti-*Ostertagia ostertagi* antibodies in individual milk samples as decision parameter for selective anthelmintic treatment in dairy cows. Prev. Vet. Med. 93 (2–3), 147–152.

Charlier, J., Van der Voort, M., Hogeveen, H., Vercruysse, J., 2012. ParaCalc®- -a novel tool to evaluate the economic importance of worm infections on the dairy farm. Vet. Parasitol. 184, 204–211.

Charlier, J., van der Voort, M., Kenyon, F., Skuce, P., Vercruysse, J., 2014. Chasing helminths and their economic impact on farmed ruminants. Trends Parasitol. 30, 361–367.

Charlier, J., Rinaldi, L., Musella, V., Ploeger, H.W., Chartier, C., Vineer, H.R., Hinney, B., von Samson-Himmelstjerna, G., Băcescu, B., Mickiewicz, M., Mateus, T.L., Martinez-Valladares, M., Quealy, S., Azaizeh, H., Sekovska, B., Akkari, H., Petkevicius, S., Hektoen, L., Höglund, J., Morgan, E.R., Bartley, D.J., Claerebout, E., 2020. Initial assessment of the economic burden of major parasitic helminth infections to the ruminant livestock industry in Europe. Prev. Vet. Med. 182, 105103.

Charlier, J., Bartley, D.J., Sotiraki, S., Martinez-Valladares, M., Claerebout, E., von Samson-Himmelstjerna, G., Thamsborg, S.M., Hoste, H., Morgan, E.R., Rinaldi, L., 2022. Anthelmintic resistance in ruminants: challenges and solutions. Adv. Parasitol. 115, 171–227.

Chaudhry, U., Miller, M., Yazwinski, T., Kaplan, R., Gilleard, J., 2014. The presence of benzimidazole resistance mutations in *Haemonchus placei* from US cattle. Vet. Parasitol. 204, 411–415.

Chaudhry, U., Redman, E.M., Abbas, M., Muthusamy, R., Ashraf, K., Gilleard, J.S., 2015a. Genetic evidence for hybridisation between *Haemonchus contortus* and *Haemonchus placei* in natural field populations and its implications for interspecies transmission of anthelmintic resistance. Int. J. Parasitol. 45, 149–159.

Chaudhry, U., Redman, E.M., Raman, M., Gilleard, J.S., 2015b. Genetic evidence for the spread of a benzimidazole resistance mutation across southern India from a single origin in the parasitic nematode *Haemonchus contortus*. Int. J. Parasitol. 45, 721–728.

Chaudhry, U., Redman, E.M., Kaplan, R., Yazwinski, T., Sargison, N., Gilleard, J.S., 2020. Contrasting patterns of isotype-1 β-tubulin allelic diversity in *Haemonchus contortus* and *Haemonchus placei* in the southern USA are consistent with a model of localised emergence of benzimidazole resistance. Vet. Parasitol. 286, 109240.

Chen, W., Yu, H., Sun, F., Ornob, A., Brisbin, R., Ganguli, A., Vemuri, V., Strzebonski, P., Cui, G., Allen, K.J., Desai, S.A., Lin, W., Nash, D.M., Hirschberg, D.L., Brooks, I., Bashir, R., Cunningham, B.T., 2017. Mobile platform for multiplexed detection and differentiation of disease-specific nucleic acid sequences, using microfluidic loop-mediated isothermal amplification and smartphone detection. Anal. Chem. 89, 11219–11226.

Chen, B., Jiang, Y., Cao, X., Liu, C., Zhang, N., Shi, D., 2021. Droplet digital PCR as an emerging tool in detecting pathogens nucleic acids in infectious diseases. Clin. Chim. Acta 517, 156–161.

Cimino, R.O., Jeun, R., Juarez, M., Cajal, P.S., Vargas, P., Echazú, A., Bryan, P.E., Nasser, J., Krolewiecki, A., Mejia, R., 2015. Identification of human intestinal parasites affecting an asymptomatic peri-urban Argentinian population using multi-parallel quantitative real-time polymerase chain reaction. Parasit. Vectors 8, 1–7.

Clayton, H.M., 1986. Ascarids: recent advances. Veterinary clinics of North America. Equine Pract. 2 (2), 313–328.

Coghlan, A., Tyagi, R., Cotton, J.A., Holroyd, N., Rosa, B.A., Tsai, I.J., Laetsch, D.R., Beech, R.N., Day, T.A., Hallsworth-Pepin, K., Ke, H.M., Kuo, T.H., Lee, T.J., Martin, J., Maizels, R.M., Mutowo, P., Ozersky, P., Parkinson, J., Reid, A.J., Rawlings, N.D., Ribeiro, D.M., Swapna, L.S., Stanley, E., Taylor, D.W., Wheeler, N.J., Zamanian, M., Zhang, X., Allan, F., Allen, J.E., Asano, K., Babayan, S.A., Bah, G., Beasley, H., Bennett, H.M., Bisset, S.A., Castillo, E., Cook, J., Cooper, P.J., Cruz-Bustos, T., Cuéllar, C., Devaney, E., Doyle, S.R., Eberhard, M.L., Emery, A., Eom, K.S., Gilleard, J.S., Gordon, D., Harcus, Y., Harsha, B., Hawdon, J.M., Hill, D.E., Hodgkinson, J., Horák, P., Howe, K.L., Huckvale, T., Kalbe, M., Kaur, G., Kikuchi, T., Koutsovoulos, G., Kumar, S., Leach, A.R., Lomax, J., Makepeace, B., Matthews, J.B., Muro, A., O'Boyle, N.M., Olson, P.D., Osuna, A., Partono, F., Pfarr, K., Rinaldi, G., Foronda, P., Rollinson, D., Samblas, M.G., Sato, H., Schnyder, M., Scholz, T., Shafie, M., Tanya, V.N., Toledo, R., Tracey, A., Urban, J.F., Wang, L.C., Zarlenga, D., Blaxter, M.L., Mitreva, M., Berriman, M., 2019. Comparative genomics of the major parasitic worms. Nat. Genet. 51, 163–174.

Cools, P., Vlaminck, J., Albonico, M., Ame, S., Ayana, M., José Antonio, B.P., Cringoli, G., Dana, D., Keiser, J., Maurelli, M.P., Maya, C., Matoso, L.F., Montresor, A., Mekonnen, Z., Mirams, G., Corrêa-Oliveira, R., Pinto, S.A., Rinaldi, L., Sayasone, S., Thomas, E., Verweij, J.J., Vercruysse, J., Levecke, B., 2019. Diagnostic performance of a single and duplicate Kato-Katz, mini-FLOTAC, $FECPAK^{G2}$ and qPCR for the detection and quantification of soil-transmitted helminths in three endemic countries. PLoS Negl. Trop. Dis. 13 (8), e0007446.

Corning, S., 2009. Equine cyathostomins: a review of biology, clinical significance and therapy. Parasit. Vectors 25 (2), S1.

Costa-Junior, L.M., Chaudhry, U.N., Silva, C.R., Sousa, D.M., Silva, N.C., Cutrim-Júnior, J.A.A., Brito, D.R.B., Sargison, N.D., 2021. Nemabiome metabarcoding reveals differences between gastrointestinal nematode species infecting co-grazed sheep and goats. Vet. Parasitol. 289, 109339.

Cox, D.D., Todd, A.C., 1962. Survey of gastrointestinal parasitism in Wisconsin dairy cattle. J. Am. Vet. Med. Assoc. 141, 706–709.

Cringoli, G., Rinaldi, L., Maurelli, M.P., Utzinger, J., 2010. FLOTAC: new multivalent techniques for qualitative and quantitative copromicroscopic diagnosis of parasites in animals and humans. Nat. Protoc. 5 (3), 503–515.

Cringoli, G., Maurelli, M.P., Levecke, B., Bosco, A., Vercruysse, J., Utzinger, J., Rinaldi, L., 2017. The mini-FLOTAC technique for the diagnosis of helminth and protozoan infections in humans and animals. Nat. Protoc. 12 (9), 1723–1732.

Cringoli, G., Amadesi, A., Maurelli, M.P., Celano, B., Piantadosi, G., Bosco, A., Ciuca, L., Cesarelli, M., Bifulco, P., Montresor, A., Rinaldi, L., 2021. The Kubic FLOTAC microscope (KFM): a new compact digital microscope for helminth egg counts. Parasitology 148 (4), 427–434.

Cruz-Rojo, M.A., Martínez-Valladares, M., Rojo-Vázquez, F.A., 2012. *Teladorsagia circumcincta* antibodies in serum and milk samples in experimentally infected lactating ewes. Vet. Parasitol. 188 (3–4), 386–390.

Das, A.K., Nayak, J., Naik, B., Pati, S.K., Pelusi, D., 2019. Computational Intelligence in Pattern Recognition: Proceedings of CIPR 2019, first ed. Springer Nature Singapore Pte Ltd, p. 1046.

Demeler, J., Krüger, N., Krücken, J., von der Heyden, V.C., Ramünke, S., Küttler, U., Miltsch, S., López Cepeda, M., Knox, M., Vercruysse, J., Geldhof, P., Harder, A., von Samson-Himmelstjerna, G., 2013a. Phylogenetic characterization of β-tubulins and development of pyrosequencing assays for benzimidazole resistance in cattle nematodes. PLoS One 8, e70212.

Demeler, J., Ramünke, S., Wolken, S., Ianiello, D., Rinaldi, L., Gahutu, J.B., Cringoli, G., von Samson-Himmelstjerna, G., Krücken, J., 2013b. Discrimination of gastrointestinal nematode eggs from crude fecal egg preparations by inhibitor-resistant conventional and real-time PCR. PLoS One 8, e61285.

Diawara, A., Drake, L.J., Suswillo, R.R., Kihara, J., Bundy, D.A.P., Scott, M.E., Halpenny, C., Stothard, J.R., Prichard, R.K., 2009. Assays to detect β-tubulin codon 200 polymorphism in *Trichuris trichiura* and *Ascaris lumbricoides*. PLoS Negl. Trop. Dis. 3 (3), e397.

Dorris, M., De Ley, P., Blaxter, M.L., 1999. Molecular analysis of nematode diversity and the evolution of parasitism. Parasitol. Today 15 (5), 188–193.

Dowdall, S.M.J., Proudman, C.J., Klei, T.R., Mair, T., Matthews, J.B., 2004. Characterisation of IgG(T) serum antibody responses to two larval antigen complexes in horses naturally- or experimentally-infected with cyathostomins. Int. J. Parasitol. 34 (1), 101–108.

El-Badry, A.A., 2009. ELISA-based coproantigen in human strongyloidiaisis: a diagnostic method correlating with worm burden. J. Egypt. Soc. Parasitol. 39 (3), 757–768.

Elghryani, N., Crispell, J., Ebrahimi, R., Krivoruchko, M., Lobaskin, V., McOwan, T., O'Connor, W., Power, E., Voisin, B., Scholz, D., de Waal, T., 2020. Preliminary evaluation of a novel, fully automated, Telenostic device for rapid field-diagnosis of cattle parasites. Parasitology 147 (11), 1249–1253.

Elmahalawy, S.T., Halvarsson, P., Skarin, M., Höglund, J., 2018. Droplet digital polymerase chain reaction (ddPCR) as a novel method for absolute quantification of major gastro-intestinal nematodes in sheep. Vet. Parasitol. 261, 1–8.

Elsemore, D.A., 2020. Antigen detection: insights into *Toxocara* and other ascarid infections in dogs and cats. Adv. Parasitol. 109, 545–559.

Elsemore, D.A., Geng, J., Flynn, L., Cruthers, L., Lucio-Forster, A., Bowman, D.D., 2014. Enzyme-linked immunosorbent assay for coproantigen detection of *Trichuris vulpis* in dogs. J. Vet. Diagn. Invest. 26 (3), 404–411.

Elsemore, D.A., Geng, J., Cote, J., Hanna, R., Lucio-Forster, A., Bowman, D.D., 2017. Enzyme-linked immunosorbent assays for coproantigen detection of *Ancylostoma caninum* and *Toxocara canis* in dogs and *Toxocara cati* in cats. J. Vet. Diagn. Invest. 29 (5), 645–653.

Entrican, G., Charlier, J., Dalton, L., Messori, S., Sharma, S., Taylor, R., Morrow, A., 2021. Construction of generic roadmaps for the strategic coordination of global research into infectious diseases of animals and zoonoses. Transbound. Emerg. Dis. 68 (3), 1513–1520.

Erali, M., Voelkerding, K.V., Wittwer, C.T., 2008. High resolution melting applications for clinical laboratory medicine. Exp. Mol. Pathol. 85 (1), 50–58.

Evans, M.J., Chaudhry, U.N., Costa-Júnior, L.M., Hamer, K., Leeson, S.R., Sargison, N.D., 2021. A 4year observation of gastrointestinal nematode egg counts, nemabiomes and the benzimidazole resistance genotypes of *Teladorsagia circumcincta* on a Scottish sheep farm. Int. J. Parasitol. 51 (5), 393–403.

Fávero, F.C., dos Santos, L.B., Araújo, F.R., d., Ramünke, S., Krücken, J., von Samson-Himmelstjerna, G., & Borges, F. de A., 2020. *Haemonchus* sp. in beef cattle in Brazil: species composition and frequency of benzimidazole resistance alleles. Prev. Vet. Med. 185, 105162.

Fernández-Rivas, G., Rivaya, B., Romaní, N., Wang, J., Alcaide, M., Matas, L., 2021. Automated parasitological diagnosis in clinical microbiology laboratories. Sci. Rep. 11 (1), 13105.

Fernández-Soto, P., Celis-Giraldo, C.T., Collar-Fernández, C., Gorgojo, Ó., Camargo, M., Muñoz, J., Salas-Coronas, J., Patarroyo, M.A., Muro, A., 2020. Strong-LAMP assay based on a Strongyloides spp.-derived partial sequence in the 18S rRNA as potential biomarker for strongyloidiasis diagnosis in human urine samples. Dis. Markers 2020. 5265198.

Feucherolles, M., Poppert, S., Utzinger, J., Becker, S.L., 2019. MALDI-TOF mass spectrometry as a diagnostic tool in human and veterinary helminthology: a systematic review. Parasit. Vectors 12 (1), 245.

Fittipaldi, M., Codony, F., Adrados, B., Camper, A.K., Morató, J., 2011. Viable real-time PCR in environmental samples: can all data be interpreted directly? Microb. Ecol. 61 (1), 7–12.

Foreyt, W.J., 2001. Veterinary Parasitology Reference Manual, fifth ed. Iowa State University Press, Ames, p. 236.

Francis, E.K., Šlapeta, J., 2022. A new diagnostic approach to fast-track and increase the accessibility of gastrointestinal nematode identification from faeces: FECPAKG2 egg nemabiome metabarcoding. Int. J. Parasitol. (S0020-7519(22)00018-2).

Francois, P., Tangomo, M., Hibbs, J., Bonetti, E.J., Boehme, C.C., Notomi, T., Perkins, M.D., Schrenzel, J., 2011. Robustness of a loop-mediated isothermal amplification reaction for diagnostic applications. FEMS Immunol. Med. Microbiol. 62 (1), 41–48.

Frey, C.F., Eicher, R., Raue, K., Strube, C., Bodmer, M., Hentrich, B., Gottstein, B., Marreros, N., 2018. Apparent prevalence of and risk factors for infection with *Ostertagia ostertagi*, *Fasciola hepatica* and *Dictyocaulus viviparus* in Swiss dairy herds. Vet. Parasitol. 250, 52–59.

Frontera, E., Serrano, F., Reina, D., Alcaide, M., Sánchez-López, J., Navarrete, I., 2003. Serological responses to *ascaris suum* adult worm antigens in Iberian finisher pigs. J. Helminthol. 77 (2), 167–172.

Fu, Y., Liu, Y., Abuzeid, A.M.I., Huang, Y., Zhou, X., He, L., Zhao, Q., Li, X., Liu, J., Ran, R., Li, G., 2019. Establishment of a tm-shift method for detection of cat-derived hookworms. Korean J. Parasitol. 57 (1), 9–15.

Fülleborn, F., 1921. Über die Wanderung von *Ascaris* und Nematoden larven im Körper und intrauterine *Ascaris* infektion. Arch. Schiffs- u. Tropenhyg 25, 146–149.

Gadahi, J.A., Wang, S., Bo, G., Ehsan, M., Yan, R.F., Song, X.K., Xu, L.X., Li, X.R., 2016. Proteomic analysis of the excretory and secretory proteins of *Haemonchus contortus* (HcESP) binding to goat PBMCs *in vivo* revealed stage-specific binding profiles. PLoS One 11 (7), 1–26.

Gandasegui, J., Grau-Pujol, B., Cambra-Pelleja, M., Escola, V., Demontis, M.A., Cossa, A., Jamine, J.C., Balaña-Fouce, R., van Lieshout, L., Muñoz, J., Martínez-Valladares, M., Munoz, J., Krolewiecki, A.J., Mwandawiro, C., Pullan, R., Mandomando, I., Valladares, M.M., Yeshaneh, W.E., Guille, R., Williams, N.A., Fernandez, M., Sarukhan, A., Marti-Soler, H., Kepha, S., Rono, M., Baptista, E., Medley, G.,

Pitt, C., Messa Junior, A., Pelleja, M.C., Demontis, M., Gelaye, W., 2021. Improving stool sample processing and pyrosequencing for quantifying benzimidazole resistance alleles in *Trichuris trichiura* and *Necator americanus* pooled eggs. Parasit. Vectors 14, 1–12.

Ganguli, A., Ornob, A., Yu, H., Damhorst, G.L., Chen, W., Sun, F., Bhuiya, A., Cunningham, B.T., Bashir, R., 2017. Hands-free smartphone-based diagnostics for simultaneous detection of zika, chikungunya, and dengue at point-of-care. Biomed. Microdevices 19 (4), 73.

Gasser, R.B., 1999. PCR-based technology in veterinary parasitology. Vet. Parasitol. 84, 229–258.

Gasser, R.B., Hoste, H., 1995. Genetic markers for closely-related parasitic nematodes. Mol. Cell. Probes 9, 315–320.

Gasser, R.B., Chilton, N.B., Hoste, H., Beveridge, I., 1993. Rapid sequencing of rDNA from single worms and eggs of parasitic helminths. Nucleic Acids Res. 21, 2525–2526.

Gasser, R.B., Chilton, N.B., Hoste, H., Stevenson, L.A., 1994. Species identification of trichostrongyle nematodes by PCR-linked RFLP. Int. J. Parasitol. 24 (2), 291–293.

Gasser, R.B., Bott, N.J., Chilton, N.B., Hunt, P., Beveridge, I., 2008. Toward practical, DNA-based diagnostic methods for parasitic nematodes of livestock — bionomic and biotechnological implications. Biotechnol. Adv. 26 (4), 325–334.

Gehlen, H., Wulke, N., Ertelt, A., Nielsen, M.K., Morelli, S., Traversa, D., Merle, R., Wilson, D., Von Samson-Himmelstjerna, G., 2020. Comparative analysis of intestinal helminth infections in colic and non-colic control equine patients. Animals 10 (10), 1–13.

George, M.M., Vatta, A.F., Howell, S.B., Storey, B.E., McCoy, C.J., Wolstenholme, A.J., Redman, E.M., Gilleard, J.S., Kaplan, R.M., 2021. Evaluation of changes in drug susceptibility and population genetic structure in *Haemonchus contortus* following worm replacement as a means to reverse the impact of multiple-anthelmintic resistance on a sheep farm. *International journal for parasitology*. Drug Resist. 15, 134–143.

Geurden, T., Smith, E.R., Vercruysse, J., Yazwinski, T., Settje, T., Nielsen, M.K., 2022. World association for the advancement of veterinary parasitology (WAAVP) guideline for the evaluation of the efficacy of anthelmintics in food-producing and companion animals: general guidelines. Vet. Parasitol. 304, 109698.

Ghafar, A., Abbas, G., King, J., Jacobson, C., Hughes, K.J., El-Hage, C., Beasley, A., Bauquier, J., Wilkes, E.J.A., Hurley, J., Cudmore, L., Carrigan, P., Tennent-Brown, B., Nielsen, M.K., Gauci, C.G., Beveridge, I., Jabbar, A., 2021. Comparative studies on faecal egg counting techniques used for the detection of gastrointestinal parasites of equines: A systematic review. Curr. Res. Parasitol. Vector Borne Dis. 1, 100046.

Ghisi, M., Kaminsky, R., Mäser, P., 2007. Phenotyping and genotyping of *Haemonchus contortus* isolates reveals a new putative candidate mutation for benzimidazole resistance in nematodes. Vet. Parasitol. 144, 313–320.

Gilleard, J.S., Redman, E., 2016. Genetic diversity and population structure of *Haemonchus contortus*. Adv. Parasitol. 93, 31–68.

Githiori, J.B., Kooyman, F.N.J., Kruitwagen, C., Ploeger, H.W., Eysker, M., 2000. Use of a 14.2 kDa recombinant *Cooperia oncophora* protein in an ELISA for herd health monitoring of nematode infections in first grazing season calves. Vet. Parasitol. 91 (1–2), 63–78.

González, I.J., Polley, S., Hopkins, H., Sutherland, C., Mori, Y., Perkins, M., Bell, D., 2012. Molecular diagnosis for screening and elimination of malaria: performance of the first commercially-available malaria LAMP test. Malar. J. 11 (Suppl 1), O30.

Gordon, H.M., Whitlock, H.V., 1939. A new technique for counting nematode eggs in sheep faeces. J. Council. Sci. Ind. Res. 12, 50–52.

Gordon, C.A., McManus, D.P., Acosta, L.P., Olveda, R.M., Williams, G.M., Ross, A.G., Gray, D.J., Gobert, G.N., 2015. Multiplex real-time PCR monitoring of intestinal helminths in humans reveals widespread polyparasitism in Northern Samar, the Philippines. Int. J. Parasitol. 45, 477–483.

Goto, Y., Akahori, R., Yanagi, I., Takeda, K., 2019. Solid-state nanopores towards single-molecule DNA sequencing. J. Hum. Genet. 65, 69–77.
Grillo, V., Jackson, F., Gilleard, J.S., 2006. Characterisation of *Teladorsagia circumcincta* microsatellites and their development as population genetic markers. Mol. Biochem. Parasitol. 148, 181–189.
Grillo, V., Craig, B.H., Wimmer, B., Gilleard, J.S., 2008. Microsatellite genotyping supports the hypothesis that *Teladorsagia davtiani* and *Teladorsagia trifurcata* are morphotypes of *Teladorsagia circumcincta*. Mol. Biochem. Parasitol. 159 (1), 59–63.
Gyawali, P., Sidhu, J.P.S., Ahmed, W., Jagals, P., Toze, S., 2015. Rapid concentration and sensitive detection of hookworm ova from wastewater matrices using a real-time PCR method. Exp. Parasitol. 159, 5–12.
Gyawali, P., Ahmed, W., Sidhu, J.P.S., Nery, S.V., Clements, A.C., Traub, R., McCarthy, J.S., Llewellyn, S., Jagals, P., Toze, S., 2016. Quantitative detection of viable helminth ova from raw wastewater, human feces, and environmental soil samples using novel PMA-qPCR methods. Environ. Sci. Pollut. Res. Int. 23, 18639–18648.
Gyawali, P., Sidhu, J.P.S., Ahmed, W., Jagals, P., Toze, S., 2017. Comparison of culture-based, vital stain and PMA-qPCR methods for the quantitative detection of viable hookworm ova. Water Sci. Technol. 75, 2615–2621.
Halvarsson, P., Höglund, J., 2021. Sheep nemabiome diversity and its response to anthelmintic treatment in Swedish sheep herds. Parasit. Vectors 14 (1), 114.
Harmon, A.F., Williams, Z.B., Holler, L.D., Hildreth, M.B., 2007a. Comparison of three different preservatives for morphological and real-time PCR analyses of *Haemonchus contortus* eggs. Vet. Parasitol. 145, 361–365.
Harmon, A.F., Williams, Z.B., Zarlenga, D.S., Hildreth, M.B., 2007b. Real-time PCR for quantifying *Haemonchus contortus* eggs and potential limiting factors. Parasitol. Res. 101, 71–76.
Hassan, N., Aboelsoued, D., Farag, T.K., Hassan, S.E., Abu El Ezz, N., 2019. Assessment of *Haemonchus contortus* larval and adult somatic antigens in sero-diagnosis of haemonchosis in naturally infected sheep and goats. J. Parasit. Dis. 43 (4), 718–725.
Hayward, A.D., 2013. Causes and consequences of intra- and inter-host heterogeneity in defence against nematodes. Parasite Immunol. 35 (11), 362–373.
Heather, J.M., Chain, B., 2016. The sequence of sequencers: the history of sequencing DNA. Genomics 107, 1–8.
Heder, M., 2017. From NASA to EU: the evolution of the TRL scale in Public Sector Innovation. Innov. J.: Public Sector Innov. J. 22 (2).
Heithoff, D.M., Barnes, L.V., Mahan, S.P., Fox, G.N., Arn, K.E., Ettinger, S.J., Bishop, A.M., Fitzgibbons, L.N., Fried, J.C., Low, D.A., Samuel, C.E., Mahan, M.J., 2022. Assessment of a smartphone-based loop-mediated isothermal amplification assay for detection of SARS-CoV-2 and influenza viruses. JAMA Netw. Open 5, e2145669.
Hendrix, C.M., 2006. Diagnostic Parasitology for Veterinary Technicians, third ed. MO, Elsevier Mosby, St. Louis, p. 285.
Hernández, J.N., Hernández, A., Stear, M.J., Conde-Felipe, M., Rodríguez, E., Piedrafita, D., González, J.F., 2016. Potential role for mucosal IgA in modulating *Haemonchus contortus* adult worm infection in sheep. Vet. Parasitol. 223, 153–158.
Hinney, B., Schoiswohl, J., Melville, L., Ameen, V.J., Wille-Piazzai, W., Bauer, K., Joachim, A., Krücken, J., Skuce, P.J., Krametter-Frötscher, R., 2020. High frequency of benzimidazole resistance alleles in trichostrongyloids from Austrian sheep flocks in an alpine transhumance management system. BMC Vet. Res. 16, 132.
Hinney, B., Wiedermann, S., Hofer, M., Bosco, A., Dimov, O., Rinaldi, L., Krücken, J., Joachim, A., Steinborn, R., 2021. Benzimidazole resistance alleles in *Haemonchus contortus* detected by digital PCR. In: 28th Conference of the World Association for the Advancement of Veterinary Parasitology. (p. O-3020).

Hoekstra, R., Criado-Fornelio, A., Fakkeldij, J., Bergman, J., Roos, M.H., 1997. Microsatellites of the parasitic nematode *Haemonchus contortus*: polymorphism and linkage with a direct repeat. Mol. Biochem. Parasitol. 89, 97–107.

Högberg, N., Hessle, A., Lidfors, L., Enweji, N., Höglund, J., 2021. Nematode parasitism affects lying time and overall activity patterns in lambs following pasture exposure around weaning. Vet. Parasitol. 296, 109500.

Höglund, J., Dahlström, F., Engström, A., Hessle, A., Jakubek, E.B., Schnieder, T., Strube, C., Sollenberg, S., 2010. Antibodies to major pasture borne helminth infections in bulk-tank milk samples from organic and nearby conventional dairy herds in south-Central Sweden. Vet. Parasitol. 171 (3–4), 293–299.

Höglund, J., Carlsson, A., Gustafsson, K., 2021. Effects of lambing season on nematode faecal egg output in ewes. Vet. Parasitol.: Reg. Stud. Rep. 26, 100633.

Holterman, M., van der Wurff, A., van den Elsen, S., van Megen, H., Bongers, T., Holovachov, O., Bakker, J., Helder, J., 2006. Phylum-wide analysis of SSU rDNA reveals deep phylogenetic relationships among nematodes and accelerated evolution toward crown clades. Mol. Biol. Evol. 23, 1792–1800.

Holzinger, A., Carrington, A., Müller, H., 2020. Measuring the quality of explanations: the system causability scale (SCS): comparing human and machine explanations. Kunstliche Intelligenz 34 (2), 193–198.

Humbert, J.F., Cabaret, J., 1995. Use of random amplified polymorphic DNA for identification of ruminant trichostrongylid nematodes. Parasitol. Res. 81 (1), 1–5.

Humbert, J.F., Cabaret, J., Elard, L., Leignel, V., Silvestre, A., 2001. Molecular approaches to studying benzimidazole resistance in trichostrongylid nematode parasites of small ruminants. Vet. Parasitol. 101, 405–414.

Hussain, T., Periasamy, K., Nadeem, A., Babar, M.E., Pichler, R., Diallo, A., 2014. Sympatric species distribution, genetic diversity and population structure of *Haemonchus* isolates from domestic ruminants in Pakistan. Vet. Parasitol. 206, 188–199.

Iamrod, K., Chaidee, A., Rucksaken, R., Kopolrat, K.Y., Worasith, C., Wongphutorn, P., Intuyod, K., Pinlaor, S., Sithithaworn, J., Sithithaworn, P., Hongsrichan, N., 2022. Development and efficacy of droplet digital PCR for detection of Strongyloides stercoralis in stool. Am. J. Trop. Med. Hyg. 106, 312–319.

Inácio, S.V., Ferreira Gomes, J., Xavier Falcão, A., Nagase Suzuki, C.T., Bertequini Nagata, W., Nery Loiola, S.H., Martins Dos Santos, B., Soares, F.A., Rosa, S.L., Baptista, C.B., Borges Alves, G., Saraiva Bresciani, K.D., 2020. Automated diagnosis of canine gastrointestinal parasites using image analysis. Pathogens (Basel, Switzerland) 9 (2), 139.

Inácio, S.V., Gomes, J.F., Falcão, A.X., Martins Dos Santos, B., Soares, F.A., Nery Loiola, S.H., Rosa, S.L., Nagase Suzuki, C.T., Bresciani, K., 2021. Automated diagnostics: advances in the diagnosis of intestinal parasitic infections in humans and animals. Front. Vet. Sci. 8, 715406.

Jack, C., Hotchkiss, E., Sargison, N.D., Toma, L., Milne, C., Bartley, D.J., 2022. Determining the influence of socio-psychological factors on the adoption of individual 'best practice' parasite control behaviours from Scottish sheep farmers. Prev. Vet. Med. 200, 105594.

Jarad, N.I., Abbas, A.K., Aάiz, N.N., 2019. Serodiagnosis of toxocariasis by ELISA test using anti- T. Canis IgG antibodies in stray dogs compared to PCR. Iraqi J. Vet. Sci. 33 (2), 367–370.

Jimenez Castro, P.D., Howell, S.B., Schaefer, J.J., Avramenko, R.W., Gilleard, J.S., Kaplan, R.M., 2019. Multiple drug resistance in the canine hookworm *Ancylostoma caninum*: an emerging threat? Parasit. Vectors 12, 576.

Jimenez Castro, P.D., Venkatesan, A., Redman, E., Chen, R., Malatesta, A., Huff, H., Zuluaga Salazar, D.A., Avramenko, R., Gilleard, J.S., Kaplan, R.M., 2021. Multiple drug resistance in hookworms infecting greyhound dogs in the USA. *International journal for parasitology*. Drug Resist. 17, 107–117.

Joachim, A., Dülmer, N., Daugschies, A., 1999. Differentiation of two *Oesophagostomum* spp. from pigs, *O. dentatum* and *O. quadrispinulatum*, by computer-assisted image analysis of fourth-stage larvae. Parasitol. Int. 48 (1), 63–71.

Joachim, A., Winkler, C., Ruczizka, U., Ladinig, A., Koch, M., Tichy, A., Schwarz, L., 2021. Comparison of different detection methods for *ascaris suum* infection on Austrian swine farms. Porc. Health Manag. 7 (1), 1–8.

Jürgenschellert, L., Krücken, J., Bousquet, E., Bartz, J., Heyer, N., Nielsen, M.K., von Samson-Himmelstjerna, G., 2022. Occurrence of strongylid nematode parasites on horse farms in Berlin and Brandenburg, Germany with high seroprevalence of *Strongylus vulgaris*. Front. Vet. Sci. 9, 892920.

Kamani, J., Massetti, L., Olubade, T., Balami, J.A., Samdi, K.M., Traub, R.J., Colella, V., González-Miguel, J., 2021. Canine gastrointestinal parasites as a potential source of zoonotic infections in Nigeria: A nationwide survey. Prev. Vet. Med. 192, 105385.

Kandil, O.M., Hendawy, S.H.M., El Namaky, A.H., Gabrashanska, M.P., Nanev, V.N., 2017. Evaluation of different *Haemonchus contortus* antigens for diagnosis of sheep haemonchosis by ELISA and their cross reactivity with other helminthes. J. Parasit. Dis. 41 (3), 678–683.

Kaplan, R.M., 2020. Biology, epidemiology, diagnosis, and Management of Anthelmintic Resistance in gastrointestinal nematodes of livestock. Vet. Clin. North Am. Food Anim. Pract. 36 (1), 17–30.

Kaplan, R.M., Levecke, B., Denwood, M., Torgerson, P.R., Dobson, R.J., Thamsborg, S.M., Nielsen, M.K., Gilleard, J.S., Vercruysse, J., 2022. World Association for the Advancement of veterinary parasitology (WAAVP) guidelines for diagnosing anthelmintic resistance using the faecal egg count reduction test in ruminants, horses and swine. Vet. Parasitol.

Karadjian, G., Bilska-Zając, E., Bahn, P., Py, J.-S., Johne, A., Gassilloud, B., Różycki, M., Cencek, T., Mayer-Scholl, A., Vallée, I., 2020. Species identification of *trichinella* originated from various host and different geographical location by MALDI-TOF. Exp. Parasitol. 213, 107890.

Karanikola, S.N., Krücken, J., Ramünke, S., de Waal, T., Höglund, J., Charlier, J., Weber, C., Müller, E., Kowalczyk, S.J., Kaba, J., von Samson-Himmelstjerna, G., Demeler, J., 2015. Development of a multiplex fluorescence immunological assay for the simultaneous detection of antibodies against *Cooperia oncophora*, *Dictyocaulus viviparus* and *Fasciola hepatica* in cattle. Parasit. Vectors 8, 335.

Kazemi, F., Arjmand, R., Fallahizadeh, S., Tavalla, M., 2020. Comparison of the detection of *Toxocara* Spp. in the soils of public Parks of Ahvaz (southwest of Iran) by PCR and loop-mediated isothermal amplification (LAMP). Infect. Disord. Drug Targets 21, 375–383.

Keegan, J.D., Good, B., De Waal, T., Fanning, J., Keane, O.M., 2017. Genetic basis of benzimidazole resistance in *Teladorsagia circumcincta* in Ireland. Ir. Vet. J. 70, 8.

Keus, A., Kloosterman, A., Van den Brink, R., 1981. Detection of antibodies to *Cooperia* ssp. and *Ostertagia* ssp. in calves with the enzyme linked immunosorbent assay (ELISA). Vet. Parasitol. 8 (3), 229–236.

Khangembam, R., Tóth, M., Vass, N., Várady, M., Czeglédi, L., Farkas, R., Antonopoulos, A., 2021. Point of care colourimetric and lateral flow LAMP assay for the detection of *Haemonchus contortus* in ruminant faecal samples. Parasite (Paris, France) 28, 82.

Khoshakhlagh, P., Spotin, A., Mahami-Oskouei, M., Shahbazi, A., Ozlati, M., 2017. Loop-mediated isothermal amplification as a reliable assay for *Toxocara canis* infection in pet dogs. Parasitol. Res. 116 (9), 2591–2597.

Kotwa, J.D., French, S.K., Greer, T., Elsemore, D.A., Hanna, R., Jardine, C.M., Pearl, D.L., Weese, J.S., Mercer, N., Peregrine, A.S., 2021. Prevalence of intestinal parasites in dogs in southern Ontario, Canada, based on fecal samples tested using sucrose double centrifugation and fecal dx® tests. Vet. Parasitol.: Reg. Stud. Rep. 26, 100618.

Kotze, A.C., Hunt, P.W., Skuce, P., von Samson-Himmelstjerna, G., Martin, R.J., Sager, H., Krücken, J., Hodgkinson, J., Lespine, A., Jex, A.R., Gilleard, J.S., Beech, R.N., Wolstenholme, A.J., Demeler, J., Robertson, A.P., Charvet, C.L., Neveu, C., Kaminsky, R., Rufener, L., Alberich, M., Menez, C., Prichard, R.K., 2014. Recent advances in candidate-gene and whole-genome approaches to the discovery of anthelmintic resistance markers and the description of drug/receptor interactions. Int. J. Parasitol. Drugs Drug Resist. 4 (3), 164–184.

Kotze, A.C., Gilleard, J.S., Doyle, S.R., Prichard, R.K., 2020. Challenges and opportunities for the adoption of molecular diagnostics for anthelmintic resistance. *International journal for parasitology*. Drug Resist. 14, 264–273.

Kouam, M.K., Ngueguim, F.D., Kantzoura, V., 2018. Internal parasites of pigs and worm control practices in Bamboutos, Western highlands of Cameroon. J. Parasitol. Res. (8242486).

Krecek, R.C., Waller, P.J., 2006. Towards the implementation of the "basket of options" approach to helminth parasite control of livestock: emphasis on the tropics/subtropics. Vet. Parasitol. 139, 270–282.

Kringel, H., Thamsborg, S.M., Petersen, H.H., Göring, H.H.H., Skallerup, P., Nejsum, P., 2015. Serum antibody responses in pigs trickle-infected with *ascaris* and *Trichuris*: Heritabilities and associations with parasitological findings. Vet. Parasitol. 211 (3–4), 306–311.

Kwa, M.S., Veenstra, J.G., Van Dijk, M., Roos, M.H., 1995. Beta-tubulin genes from the parasitic nematode *Haemonchus contortus* modulate drug resistance in *Caenorhabditis elegans*. J. Mol. Biol. 246, 500–510.

Lagatie, O., Verheyen, A., Van Hoof, K., Lauwers, D., Odiere, M.R., Vlaminck, J., Levecke, B., Stuyver, L.J., 2020. Detection of *Ascaris lumbricoides* infection by aba-1 coproantigen elisa. PLoS Negl. Trop. Dis. 14 (10), e0008807.

Lane, C., 1924. The mass diagnosis of ankylostome infestation. (parts II toVII.). Trans. R. Soc. Trop. Med. Hyg. 17, 407–436.

Lassen, B., Geldhof, P., Hälli, O., Vlaminck, J., Oliviero, C., Orro, T., Heinonen, M., 2019. Anti-*ascaris suum* IgG antibodies in fattening pigs with different respiratory conditions. Vet. Parasitol. 265, 85–90.

Learmount, J., Conyers, C., Hird, H., Morgan, C., Craig, B.H., von Samson-Himmelstjerna, G., Taylor, M., 2009. Development and validation of real-time PCR methods for diagnosis of *Teladorsagia circumcincta* and *Haemonchus contortus* in sheep. Vet. Parasitol. 166 (3–4), 268–274.

Learmount, J., Stephens, N., Boughtflower, V., Barrecheguren, A., Rickell, K., Massei, G., Taylor, M., 2016. Three-year evaluation of best practice guidelines for nematode control on commercial sheep farms in the UK. Vet. Parasitol. 226, 116–123.

Levecke, B., Dobson, R.J., Speybroeck, N., Vercruysse, J., Charlier, J., 2012. Novel insights in the faecal egg count reduction test for monitoring drug efficacy against gastrointestinal nematodes of veterinary importance. Vet. Parasitol. 188 (3–4), 391–396.

Li, H., Bai, R., Zhao, Z., Tao, L., Ma, M., Ji, Z., Jian, M., Ding, Z., Dai, X., Bao, F., Liu, A., 2018. Application of droplet digital PCR to detect the pathogens of infectious diseases. Biosci. Rep. 38 (6) (BSR20181170).

Li, Y., Zheng, R., Wu, Y., Chu, K., Xu, Q., Sun, M., Smith, Z.J., 2019. A low-cost, automated parasite diagnostic system via a portable, robotic microscope and deep learning. J. Biophotonics 12 (9), e201800410.

Lichtenfels, J.R., Hoberg, E.P., Zarlenga, D.S., 1997. Systematics of gastrointestinal nematodes of domestic ruminants: advances between 1992 and 1995 and proposals for future research. Vet. Parasitol. 72 (3–4), 225–245.

Lindgren, K., Gunnarsson, S., Höglund, J., Lindahl, C., Roepstorff, A., 2020. Nematode parasite eggs in pasture soils and pigs on organic farms in Sweden. Org. Agric. 10, 289–300.

Little, S.E., Barrett, A.W., Beall, M.J., Bowman, D.D., Dangoudoubiyam, S., Elsemore, D.A., Liotta, J., Lucio-Forster, A., McCrann, D.J., Snowden, K.F., Starkey, L.A., Tasse, S., 2019. Coproantigen detection augments diagnosis of common nematode infections in dogs. Top. Companion Anim. Med. 35, 42–46.

Ljungström, S., Melville, L., Skuce, P.J., Höglund, J., 2018. Comparison of four diagnostic methods for detection and relative quantification of *Haemonchus contortus* eggs in feces samples. Front. Vet. Sci. 4, 239.

Llewellyn, S., Inpankaew, T., Nery, S.V., Gray, D.J., Verweij, J.J., Clements, A.C.A., Gomes, S.J., Traub, R., McCarthy, J.S., 2016. Application of a multiplex quantitative PCR to assess prevalence and intensity of intestinal parasite infections in a controlled clinical trial. PLoS Negl. Trop. Dis. 10, e0004380.

Lu, Q., Liu, G., Xiao, C., Hu, C., Zhang, S., Xu, R.X., Chu, K., Xu, Q., Smith, Z.J., 2018. A modular, open-source, slide-scanning microscope for diagnostic applications in resource-constrained settings. PLoS One 13 (3), e0194063.

Macuhova, K., Kumagai, T., Akao, N., Ohta, N., 2010. Loop-mediated isothermal amplification assay for detection and discrimination of *Toxocara canis* and *Toxocara cati* eggs directly from sand samples. J. Parasitol. 96, 1224–1227.

MAFF, 1986. Manual of Veterinary Parasitological Laboratory Techniques. Her Majesty's Stationary Office, London, UK.

Malama, E., Hoffmann-Köhler, P., Biedermann, I., Koopmann, R., Krücken, J., Molina, J.M., Moreno, A.M., von Samson-Himmelstjerna, G., Sotiraki, S., Demeler, J., 2014. Development of a milk and serum ELISA test for the detection of *Teladorsagia circumcincta* antibodies in goats using experimentally and naturally infected animals. Parasitol. Res. 113 (10), 3651–3660.

Martin, F., Halvarsson, P., Delhomme, N., Höglund, J., Tydén, E., 2021. Exploring the β-tubulin gene family in a benzimidazole-resistant *Parascaris univalens* population. *International journal for parasitology*. Drug Resist. 17, 84–91.

Martínez-Pérez, J.M., Vandekerckhove, E., Vlaminck, J., Geldhof, P., Martínez-Valladares, M., 2017. Serological detection of *ascaris suum* at fattening pig farms is linked with performance and management indices. Vet. Parasitol. 248, 33–38.

Martínez-Valladares, M., Vara-Del Río, M.P., Cruz-Rojo, M.A., Rojo-Vázquez, F.A., 2005. Genetic resistance to *Teladorsagia circumcincta*: IgA and parameters at slaughter in Churra sheep. Parasite Immunol. 27 (6), 213–218.

Martínez-Valladares, M., Donnan, A., Geldhof, P., Jackson, F., Rojo-Vázquez, F.A., Skuce, P., 2012. Pyrosequencing analysis of the beta-tubulin gene in Spanish *Teladorsagia circumcincta* field isolates. Vet. Parasitol. 184, 371–376.

Martínez-Valladares, M., Valderas-García, E., Gandasegui, J., Skuce, P., Morrison, A., De Agüero, C.G., V., Cambra-Pellejà, M., Balaña-Fouce, R., & Rojo-Vázquez, F.A., 2020. *Teladorsagia circumcincta* beta tubulin: the presence of the E198L polymorphism on its own is associated with benzimidazole resistance. Parasit. Vectors 13, 453.

Massetti, L., Colella, V., Zendejas, P.A., Ng-Nguyen, D., Harriott, L., Marwedel, L., Wiethoelter, A., Traub, R.J., 2020. High-throughput multiplex qPCRs for the surveillance of zoonotic species of canine hookworms. PLoS Negl. Trop. Dis. 14, e0008392.

Massetti, L., Kamani, J., Wiethoelter, A., McDonagh, P., Colella, V., Traub, R.J., 2021. Field application of a novel multiplex qPCR assay reveals the occurrence of the zoonotic hookworm *Ancylostoma braziliense* in Nigerian dogs. Acta Trop. 213, 105758.

Matthews, J.B., 2008. An update on cyathostomins: anthelmintic resistance and worm control. Equine Vet. Educ. 20 (10), 552–560.

Matthews, J.B., Geldhof, P., Tzelos, T., Claerebout, E., 2016. Progress in the development of subunit vaccines for gastrointestinal nematodes of ruminants. Parasite Immunol. 38 (12), 744–753.

Maurelli, M.P., Amadesi, A., Sansone, C., Marrone, S., Gravina, M., Bosco, A., Celano, B., Rinaldi, L., Cringoli, G., 2021. The Kubic FLOTAC microscope: a new tool for helminth eggs diagnosis in veterinary and human field. In: *Proceeding of XXXI National Congress of Italian Society of Parasitology (SOIPA) & 2021 ESDA EVENT Teramo, Italy, 16–19 June 2021*. pp. 233.
Maurelli, M.P., Dourado Martins, O.M., Morgan, E.R., Charlier, J., Cringoli, G., Mateus, T.L., Bacescu, B., Chartier, C., Claerebout, E., de Waal, T., Helm, C., Hertzberg, H., Hinney, B., Höglund, J., Kyriánová, I.A., Mickiewicz, M., Petkevičius, S., Simin, S., Sotiraki, S., Tosheska, M., Toth, M., Martínez-Valladares, M., Varady, M., Sekovska, B., von Samson-Himmelstjerna, G., Rinaldi, L., 2020. A qualitative market analysis applied to mini-FLOTAC and fill-FLOTAC for diagnosis of helminth infections in ruminants. Front. Vet. Sci. 22 (7), 580649.
Maurelli, M.P., Pepe, P., Illiano, S., Nocerino, M., Ciuca, L., Saralli, G., Cringoli, G., Rinaldi, L., 2022. A five-year retrospective study on ascarid infections in dogs in southern Italy. Fünfjährige retrospektive Studie zu Askarideninfektionen bei Hunden in Süditalien. Schweiz. Arch. Tierheilkd. 164 (1), 79–88.
Mayer-Scholl, A., Murugaiyan, J., Neumann, J., Bahn, P., Reckinger, S., Nöckler, K., 2016. Rapid identification of the foodborne pathogen *trichinella* spp. by matrix-assisted laser desorption/ionization mass spectrometry. PLoS One 11, e0152062.
McBean, D., Nath, M., Kenyon, F., Zile, K., Bartley, D.J., Jackson, F., 2016. Faecal egg counts and immune markers in a line of Scottish cashmere goats selected for resistance to gastrointestinal nematode parasite infection. Vet. Parasitol. 229, 1–8.
McNally, J., Callan, D., Andronicos, N., Bott, N., Hunt, P.W., 2013. DNA-based methodology for the quantification of gastrointestinal nematode eggs in sheep faeces. Vet. Parasitol. 198, 325–335.
McWilliam, H.E.G., Nisbet, A.J., Dowdall, S.M.J., Hodgkinson, J.E., Matthews, J.B., 2010. Identification and characterisation of an immunodiagnostic marker for cyathostomin developing stage larvae. Int. J. Parasitol. 40 (3), 265–275.
Mejia, R., Vicuña, Y., Broncano, N., Sandoval, C., Vaca, M., Chico, M., Cooper, P.J., Nutman, T.B., 2013. A novel, multi-parallel, real-time polymerase chain reaction approach for eight gastrointestinal parasites provides improved diagnostic capabilities to resource-limited at-risk populations. Am. J. Trop. Med. Hyg. 88, 1041–1047.
Melville, L., Kenyon, F., Javed, S., McElarney, I., Demeler, J., Skuce, P., 2014. Development of a loop-mediated isothermal amplification (LAMP) assay for the sensitive detection of *Haemonchus contortus* eggs in ovine faecal samples. Vet. Parasitol. 206, 308–312.
Melville, L.A., Redman, E., Morrison, A.A., Rebecca Chen, P.C., Avramenko, R., Mitchell, S., Van Dijk, J., Innocent, G., Sargison, F., Aitken, C., Gilleard, J.S., Bartley, D.J., 2020. Large scale screening for benzimidazole resistance mutations in *Nematodirus battus*, using both pyrosequence genotyping and deep amplicon sequencing, indicates the early emergence of resistance on UK sheep farms. *International journal for parasitology*. Drug Resist. 12, 68–76.
Merlin, A., Shaw, R., Chauvin, A., Bareille, N., Chartier, C., 2017. Significance of anti-CarLA salivary IgA antibody in first grazing season cattle naturally infected with gastrointestinal nematodes. Vet. Parasitol. 243, 36–41.
Mes, T.H., Ploeger, H.W., Terlou, M., Kooyman, F.N., Van der Ploeg, M.P., Eysker, M., 2001. A novel method for the isolation of gastro-intestinal nematode eggs that allows automated analysis of digital images of egg preparations and high throughput screening. Parasitology 123 (Pt 3), 309–314.
Mes, T.H., Eysker, M., Ploeger, H.W., 2007. A simple, robust and semi-automated parasite egg isolation protocol. Nat. Protoc. 2 (3), 486–489.
Meshgi, B., Jalousian, F., Masih, Z., 2015. Phylogenetic study of *Haemonchus* species from Iran based on morpho-molecular characterization. Iran. J. Parasitol. 10 (2), 189–196.

Mirams, G., 2016. FECPAK^{G2} is a novel online faecal egg counting system for either remote location or laboratory/clinic based parasite FEC diagnostics. In: Proceedings of the Society of Sheep and Beef Cattle Veterinarians of the New Zealand Veterinary Association, pp. 65–69.
Mitani, Y., Lezhava, A., Kawai, Y., Kikuchi, T., Oguchi-Katayama, A., Kogo, Y., Itoh, M., Miyagi, T., Takakura, H., Hoshi, K., Kato, C., Arakawa, T., Shibata, K., Fukui, K., Masui, R., Kuramitsu, S., Kiyotani, K., Chalk, A., Tsunekawa, K., Murakami, M., Kamataki, T., Oka, T., Shimada, H., Cizdziel, P.E., Hayashizaki, Y., 2007. Rapid SNP diagnostics using asymmetric isothermal amplification and a new mismatch-suppression technology. Nat. Methods 4, 257–262.
Mitchell, M.C., Tzelos, T., Handel, I., McWilliam, H.E.G., Hodgkinson, J.E., Nisbet, A.J., Kharchenko, V.O., Burgess, S.T.G., Matthews, J.B., 2016. Development of a recombinant protein-based ELISA for diagnosis of larval cyathostomin infection. Parasitology 143 (8), 1055–1066.
Mitchell, C.J., O'Sullivan, C.M., Pinloche, E., Wilkinson, T., Morphew, R.M., McEwan, N.R., 2019. Using next-generation sequencing to determine diversity of horse intestinal worms: identifying the equine "nemabiome". J. Equine Sci. 30, 1–5.
Mohammadi, M.M., Bavi, O., 2021. DNA sequencing: an overview of solid-state and biological nanopore-based methods. Biophys. Rev. 14, 99–110.
Mohammedsalih, K.M., Krücken, J., Khalafalla, A., Bashar, A., Juma, F.-R., Abakar, A., Abdalmalaik, A.A.H., Coles, G., von Samson-Himmelstjerna, G., 2020. New codon 198 β-tubulin polymorphisms in highly benzimidazole resistant *Haemonchus contortus* from goats in three different states in Sudan. Parasit. Vectors 13, 114.
Mohammedsalih, K.M., Krücken, J., Bashar, A., Juma, F.-R., Abdalmalaik, A.A.H., Khalafalla, A., Abakar, A., Coles, G., von Samson-Himmelstjerna, G., 2021. Susceptible trichostrongyloid species mask presence of benzimidazole-resistant *Haemonchus contortus* in cattle. Parasit. Vectors 14, 101.
Montresor, A., Mupfasoni, D., Mikhailov, A., Mwinzi, P., Lucianez, A., Jamsheed, M., Gasimov, E., Warusavithana, S., Yajima, A., Bisoffi, Z., Buonfrate, D., Steinmann, P., Utzinger, J., Levecke, B., Vlaminck, J., Cools, P., Vercruysse, J., Cringoli, G., Rinaldi, L., Blouin, B., Gyorkos, T.W., 2020. The global progress of soil-transmitted helminthiases control in 2020 and World Health Organization targets for 2030. PLoS Negl. Trop. Dis. 14 (8), e0008505.
Morgan, E.R., Lanusse, C., Rinaldi, L., Charlier, J., Vercruysse, J., 2022. Confounding factors affecting faecal egg count reduction as a measure of anthelmintic efficacy. Facteurs de confusion affectant la réduction du nombre d'œufs fécaux comme mesure de l'efficacité anthelminthique. Parasite (Paris, France) 29, 20.
Moser, W., Bärenbold, O., Mirams, G.J., Cools, P., Vlaminck, J., Ali, S.M., Ame, S.M., Hattendorf, J., Vounatsou, P., Levecke, B., Keiser, J., 2018. Diagnostic comparison between FECPAK^{G2} and the Kato-Katz method for analyzing soil-transmitted helminth eggs in stool. PLoS Negl. Trop. Dis. 12 (6), e0006562.
Mugambi, R.M., Agola, E.L., Mwangi, I.N., Kinyua, J., Shiraho, E.A., Mkoji, G.M., 2015. Development and evaluation of a loop mediated isothermal amplification (LAMP) technique for the detection of hookworm (*Necator americanus*) infection in fecal samples. Parasit. Vectors 8, 574.
Mullis, K., Faloona, F., Scharf, S., Saiki, R., Horn, G., Erlich, H., 1986. Specific enzymatic amplification of DNA *in vitro*: the polymerase Chain reaction. Cold Spring Harb. Symp. Quant. Biol. 51 (Pt 1), 263–273.
Nagamori, Y., Hall Sedlak, R., DeRosa, A., Pullins, A., Cree, T., Loenser, M., Larson, B.S., Smith, R.B., Goldstein, R., 2020. Evaluation of the VETSCAN IMAGYST: an in-clinic canine and feline fecal parasite detection system integrated with a deep learning algorithm. Parasit. Vectors 13 (1), 346.

Nagamori, Y., Sedlak, R.H., DeRosa, A., Pullins, A., Cree, T., Loenser, M., Larson, B.S., Smith, R.B., Penn, C., Goldstein, R., 2021. Further evaluation and validation of the VETSCAN IMAGYST: in-clinic feline and canine fecal parasite detection system integrated with a deep learning algorithm. Parasit. Vectors 14 (1), 89.

Nansen, P., Roepstorff, A., 1999. Parasitic helminths of the pig: factors influencing transmission and infection levels. Int. J. Parasitol. 29 (6), 877–891.

Naqvi, M.A., Naqvi, S.Z., Memon, M.A., Aimulajiang, K., Haseeb, M., Xu, L., Song, X., Li, X., Yan, R., 2019. Combined use of indirect ELISA and Western blotting with recombinant hepatocellular carcinoma-associated antigen 59 is a potential immunodiagnostic tool for the detection of prepatent *Haemonchus contortus* infection in goat. Animals 9 (8), 548.

Naqvi, M.A., Jamil, T., Naqvi, S.Z., Memon, M.A., Aimulajiang, K., Aleem, M.T., Ehsan, M., Xu, L., Song, X., Li, X., Yan, R., 2020. Immunodiagnostic potential of recombinant tropomyosin during prepatent *Haemonchus contortus* infection in goat. Res. Vet. Sci. 128, 197–204.

Newton, L.A., Chilton, N.B., Beveridge, I., Hoste, H., Nansen, P., Gasser, R.B., 1998. Genetic markers for strongylid nematodes of livestock defined by PCR-based restriction analysis of spacer rDNA. Acta Trop. 69, 1–15.

Ngari, M.G., Mwangi, I.N., Njoroge, M.P., Kinyua, J., Osuna, F.A., Kimeu, B.M., Okanya, P.W., Agola, E.L., 2020. Development and evaluation of a loop-mediated isothermal amplification (LAMP) diagnostic test for detection of whipworm, *Trichuris trichiura*, in faecal samples. J. Helminthol. 94, e142.

Ngui, R., Lim, Y.A.L., Chua, K.H., 2012. Rapid detection and identification of human hookworm infections through high resolution melting (HRM) analysis. PLoS One 7, e41996.

Nielsen, M.K., 2021. What makes a good fecal egg count technique? Vet. Parasitol. 296, 109509.

Nielsen, M.K., Peterson, D.S., Monrad, J., Thamsborg, S.M., Olsen, S.N., Kaplan, R.M., 2008. Detection and semi-quantification of *Strongylus vulgaris* DNA in equine faeces by real-time quantitative PCR. Int. J. Parasitol. 38, 443–453.

Nielsen, M.K., Olsen, S.N., Lyons, E.T., Monrad, J., Thamsborg, S.M., 2012. Real-time PCR evaluation of *Strongylus vulgaris* in horses on farms in Denmark and Central Kentucky. Vet. Parasitol. 190, 461–466.

Nielsen, M.K., Vidyashankar, A.N., Gravatte, H.S., Bellaw, J., Lyons, E.T., Andersen, U.V., 2014. Development of *Strongylus vulgaris*-specific serum antibodies in naturally infected foals. Vet. Parasitol. 200 (3–4), 265–270.

Nielsen, M.K., Vidyashankar, A.N., Bellaw, J., Gravatte, H.S., Cao, X., Rubinson, E.F., Reinemeyer, C.R., 2015. Serum *Strongylus vulgaris*-specific antibody responses to anthelmintic treatment in naturally infected horses. Parasitol. Res. 114 (2), 445–451.

Nielsen, M.K., Jacobsen, S., Olsen, S.N., Bousquet, E., Pihl, T., 2016. Nonstrangulating intestinal infarction associated with *Strongylus vulgaris* in referred Danish equine cases. Equine Vet. J. 48 (3), 376–379.

Nielsen, M.K., Mittel, L., Grice, A., Erskine, M., Graves, E., Vaala, W., Tully, R.C., French, D.D., Bowman, R., Kaplan, R.M., 2019. AAEP parasite control guidelines. (https://aaep.org/sites/default/files/Guidelines/AAEPParasiteControlGuidelines_0.pdf).

Nielsen, M.K., Doran, D., Slusarewicz, P., 2021. Effects of sample homogenizing on the performance of an automated strongylid egg counting system. Vet. Parasitol. 300, 109623.

Niesters, H.G.M., 2004. Molecular and diagnostic clinical virology in real time. Clin. Microbiol. Infect. 10, 5–11.

Oliveira-Arbex, A.P., David, E.B., Oliveira-Sequeira, T.C.G., Katagiri, S., Coradi, S.T., Guimarães, S., 2016. Molecular identification of *Ancylostoma* species from dogs and an assessment of zoonotic risk in low-income households, São Paulo state, Brazil. J. Helminthol. 91, 14–19.

Osaku, D., Cuba, C.F., Suzuki, C., Gomes, J.F., Falcão, A.X., 2020. Automated diagnosis of intestinal parasites: A new hybrid approach and its benefits. Comput. Biol. Med. 123, 103917.

Özben, M., von Samson-Himmelstjerna, G., Freiin von Streit, M., Wilkes, E., Hughes, K.J., Krücken, J., 2022. Absence of polymorphisms in codons 167, 198 and 200 of all seven β-tubulin isotypes of benzimidazole susceptible and resistant *Parascaris* spp. specimens from Australia. *Pathogens* (Basel Switzerland) 11 (5), 490.

Papaiakovou, M., Pilotte, N., Grant, J.R., Traub, R.J., Llewellyn, S., McCarthy, J.S., Krolewiecki, A.J., Cimino, R., Mejia, R., Williams, S.A., 2017. A novel, species-specific, real-time PCR assay for the detection of the emerging zoonotic parasite *Ancylostoma ceylanicum* in human stool. PLoS Negl. Trop. Dis. 11, e0005734.

Papaiakovou, M., Littlewood, D., Doyle, S.R., Gasser, R.B., Cantacessi, C., 2022. Worms and bugs of the gut: the search for diagnostic signatures using barcoding, and metagenomics-metabolomics. Parasit. Vectors 15 (1), 118.

Patrelle, C., Ferté, H., Jouet, D., 2014. Identification of Chabertiidae (Nematoda, Strongylida) by PCR-RFLP based method: a new diagnostic tool for cross transmission investigation between domestic and wild ruminants in France. Infect. Genet. Evol. 28, 15–20.

Peanasky, R.J., Bentz, Y., Paulson, B., Graham, D.L., Babinf, D.R., Hogan, B.J., 1984. The lsoinhibitors of chymotrypsin / elastase from *ascaris lumbricoicies* Isolation by affinity chromatography and association with the Enzymes' s2 with the technical in as- Laskowski (2) completely separated the continuous-flow paper curtain electroph. Arch. Biochem. Biophys. 232 (1), 127–134.

Pecson, B.M., Barrios, J.A., Johnson, D.R., Nelson, K.L., 2006. A real-time PCR method for quantifying viable *ascaris* eggs using the first internally transcribed spacer region of ribosomal DNA. Appl. Environ. Microbiol. 72, 7864–7872.

Pernthaner, A., Cole, S.A., Morrison, L., Green, R., Shaw, R.J., Hein, W.R., 2006. Cytokine and antibody subclass responses in the intestinal lymph of sheep during repeated experimental infections with the nematode parasite *Trichostrongylus colubriformis*. Vet. Immunol. Immunopathol. 114 (1–2), 135–148.

Pichler, R., Silbermayr, K., Periasamy, K., 2017. A novel snapback primer probe assay for the detection and discrimination of sympatric *Haemonchus* species using DNA melting analysis. Vet. Parasitol. 237, 94–103.

Pilotte, N., Papaiakovou, M., Grant, J.R., Bierwert, L.A., Llewellyn, S., McCarthy, J.S., Williams, S.A., 2016. Improved PCR-based detection of soil transmitted helminth infections using a next-generation sequencing approach to assay design. PLoS Negl. Trop. Dis. 10, e0004578.

Pilotte, N., Maasch, J.R.M.A., Easton, A.V., Dahlstrom, E., Nutman, T.B., Williams, S.A., 2019. Targeting a highly repeated germline DNA sequence for improved real-time PCR-based detection of *ascaris* infection in human stool. PLoS Negl. Trop. Dis. 13, e0007593.

Pitaksakulrat, O., Chaiyasaeng, M., Artchayasawat, A., Eamudomkarn, C., Boonmars, T., Kopolrat, K.Y., Prasopdee, S., Petney, T.N., Blair, D., Sithithaworn, P., 2021. Genetic diversity and population structure of *Haemonchus contortus* in goats from Thailand. Infect. Genet. Evol. 95, 105021.

Ploeger, H.W., Kloosterman, A., Rietveld, F.W., 1995. Acquired immunity against *Cooperia* spp. and *Ostertagia* spp. in calves: effect of level of exposure and timing of the midsummer increase. Vet. Parasitol. 58 (1–2), 61–74.

Poissant, J., Gavriliuc, S., Bellaw, J., Redman, E.M., Avramenko, R.W., Robinson, D., Workentine, M.L., Shury, T.K., Jenkins, E.J., McLoughlin, P.D., Nielsen, M.K., Gilleard, J.S., 2021. A repeatable and quantitative DNA metabarcoding assay to characterize mixed strongyle infections in horses. Int. J. Parasitol. 51, 183–192.

Poot, J., Kooyman, F.N., Dop, P.Y., Schallig, H.D., Eysker, M., Cornelissen, A.W., 1997. Use of cloned excretory/secretory low-molecular-weight proteins of *Cooperia oncophora* in a serological assay. J. Clin. Microbiol. 35 (7), 1728–1733.

Portanier, E., Garel, M., Devillard, S., Duhayer, J., Poirel, M.-T., Henri, H., Régis, C., Maillard, D., Redman, E., Itty, C., Michel, P., Bourgoin, G., 2019. Does host socio-spatial behavior lead to a fine-scale spatial genetic structure in its associated parasites? Parasite 26, 64.

Prichard, R., 1997. Application of molecular biology in veterinary parasitology. Vet. Parasitol. 71, 155–175.

Queiroz, C., Levy, M., Avramenko, R., Redman, E., Kearns, K., Swain, L., Silas, H., Uehlinger, F., Gilleard, J.S., 2020. The use of ITS-2 rDNA nemabiome metabarcoding to enhance anthelmintic resistance diagnosis and surveillance of ovine gastrointestinal nematodes. *International journal for parasitology*. Drug Resist. 14, 105–117.

Rådström, P., Knutsson, R., Wolffs, P., Lövenklev, M., Löfström, C., 2004. Pre-PCR processing : strategies to generate PCR-compatible samples. Mol. Biotechnol. 26, 133–146.

Ramünke, S., Melville, L., Rinaldi, L., Hertzberg, H., de Waal, T., von Samson-Himmelstjerna, G., Cringoli, G., Mavrot, F., Skuce, P., Krücken, J., Demeler, J., 2016. Benzimidazole resistance survey for *Haemonchus*, *Teladorsagia* and *Trichostrongylus* in three European countries using pyrosequencing including the development of new assays for *Trichostrongylus*. *International journal for parasitology*. Drug Resist. 6, 230–240.

Ramünke, S., De Almeida Borges, F., Von Son-De Fernex, E., Von Samson-Himmelstjerna, G., Krücken, J., 2018. Molecular marker sequences of cattle *Cooperia* species identify *Cooperia spatulata* as a morphotype of *Cooperia punctata*. PLoS One 13, e0200390.

Rashid, M.H., Stevenson, M.A., Waenga, S., Mirams, G., Campbell, A., Vaughan, J.L., Jabbar, A., 2018. Comparison of McMaster and FECPAK^{G2} methods for counting nematode eggs in the faeces of alpacas. Parasit. Vectors 11 (1), 278.

Rashwan, N., Bourguinat, C., Keller, K., Gunawardena, N.K., de Silva, N., Prichard, R., 2016. Isothermal diagnostic assays for monitoring single nucleotide polymorphisms in *Necator americanus* associated with benzimidazole drug resistance. PLoS Negl. Trop. Dis. 10, e0005113.

Rashwan, N., Diawara, A., Scott, M.E., Prichard, R.K., 2017a. Isothermal diagnostic assays for the detection of soil-transmitted helminths based on the SmartAmp2 method. Parasit. Vectors 10, 496.

Rashwan, N., Scott, M., Prichard, R., 2017b. Rapid genotyping of β-tubulin polymorphisms in *Trichuris trichiura* and *Ascaris lumbricoides*. PLoS Negl. Trop. Dis. 11, e0005205.

Ravindran, V.B., Shahsavari, E., Soni, S.K., Ball, A.S., 2019. Viability determination of *ascaris* ova in raw wastewater: A comparative evaluation of culture-based, BacLight live/dead staining and PMA-qPCR methods. Water Sci. Technol. 80, 817–826.

Redman, E., Whitelaw, F., Tait, A., Burgess, C., Bartley, Y., Skuce, P.J., Jackson, F., Gilleard, J.S., 2015. The emergence of resistance to the benzimidazole anthlemintics in parasitic nematodes of livestock is characterised by multiple independent hard and soft selective sweeps. PLoS Negl. Trop. Dis. 9 (2), e0003494.

Redman, E., Queiroz, C., Bartley, D.J., Levy, M., Avramenko, R.W., Gilleard, J.S., 2019. Validation of ITS-2 rDNA nemabiome sequencing for ovine gastrointestinal nematodes and its application to a large scale survey of UK sheep farms. Vet. Parasitol. 275, 108933.

Regis, S.C.S., Mendonça, L.R., dos Santos Silva, N., Dattoli, V.C.C., Alcântara-Neves, N.M., Barrouin-Melo, S.M., 2011. Seroprevalence and risk factors for canine toxocariasis by detection of specific IgG as a marker of infection in dogs from Salvador, Brazil. Acta Trop. 120 (1–2), 46–51.

Reigate, C., Evans, S., Turnbull, F., Thomas, E., 2022. Validation of the image-based FECPAKG2 system for counting sheep nematode eggs with a sensitivity of 5 epg. In: Proceeding of the Final COMBAR Conference, Athens, Greece.

Reinemeyer, C.R., Nielsen, M.K., 2009. Parasitism and colic. Vet. Clin. North Am. Equine Pract. 25 (2), 233–245.

Reslova, N., Skorpikova, L., Kyrianova, I.A., Vadlejch, J., Höglund, J., Skuce, P., Kasny, M., 2021. The identification and semi-quantitative assessment of gastrointestinal nematodes in faecal samples using multiplex real-time PCR assays. Parasit. Vectors 14, 391.

Rinaldi, L., Amadesi, A., Dufourd, E., Bosco, A., Gadanho, M., Lehebel, A., Maurelli, M.P., Chauvin, A., Charlier, J., Cringoli, G., Ravinet, N., Chartier, C., 2019. Rapid assessment of faecal egg count and faecal egg count reduction through composite sampling in cattle. Parasit. Vectors 12 (1), 353.

Rivero, J., Zurita, A., Cutillas, C., Callejón, R., 2022. The use of MALDI-TOF MS as a diagnostic tool for adult *Trichuris* species. Front. Vet. Sci. 9, 867919.

Roeber, F., Jex, A.R., Campbell, A.J.D., Campbell, B.E., Anderson, G.A., Gasser, R.B., 2011. Evaluation and application of a molecular method to assess the composition of strongylid nematode populations in sheep with naturally acquired infections. Infect. Genet. Evol. 11, 849–854.

Roeber, F., Jex, A.R., Campbell, A.J.D., Nielsen, R., Anderson, G.A., Stanley, K.K., Gasser, R.B., 2012a. Establishment of a robotic, high-throughput platform for the specific diagnosis of gastrointestinal nematode infections in sheep. Int. J. Parasitol. 42, 1151–1158.

Roeber, F., Larsen, J.W.A., Anderson, N., Campbell, A.J.D., Anderson, G.A., Gasser, R.B., Jex, A.R., 2012b. A molecular diagnostic tool to replace larval culture in conventional faecal egg count reduction testing in sheep. PLoS One 7, e37327.

Roeber, F., Hassan, E.B., Skuce, P., Morrison, A., Claerebout, E., Casaert, S., Homer, D.R., Firestone, S., Stevenson, M., Smith, L., Larsen, J., 2017a. An automated, multiplex-tandem PCR platform for the diagnosis of gastrointestinal nematode infections in cattle: an Australian-European validation study. Vet. Parasitol. 239, 62–75.

Roeber, F., Morrison, A., Casaert, S., Smith, L., Claerebout, E., Skuce, P., 2017b. Multiplexed-tandem PCR for the specific diagnosis of gastrointestinal nematode infections in sheep: an European validation study. Parasit. Vectors 10, 226.

Roepstorff, A., 1998. Natural *ascaris suum* infections in swine diagnosed by coprological and serological (ELISA) methods. Parasitol. Res. 84 (7), 537–543.

Rojas, A., Segev, G., Markovics, A., Aroch, I., Baneth, G., 2017. Detection and quantification of *Spirocerca lupi* by HRM qPCR in fecal samples from dogs with spirocercosis. Parasit. Vectors 10, 435.

Roldán, W.H., Espinoza, Y.A., 2009. Evaluation of an enzyme-linked immunoelectrotransfer blot test for the confirmatory serodiagnosis of human toxocariasis. Mem. Inst. Oswaldo Cruz 104 (3), 411–418.

Roose, S., Avramenko, R.W., Pollo, S.M.J., Wasmuth, J.D., Ame, S., Ayana, M., Betson, M., Cools, P., Dana, D., Jones, B.P., Mekonnen, Z., Morosetti, A., Venkatesan, A., Vlaminck, J., Workentine, M.L., Levecke, B., Gilleard, J.S., Geldhof, P., 2021. Characterization of the β-tubulin gene family in *Ascaris lumbricoides* and *ascaris suum* and its implication for the molecular detection of benzimidazole resistance. PLoS Negl. Trop. Dis. 15, e0009777.

Roussel, C., Drake, J., Ariza, J.M., 2019. French national survey of dog and cat owners on the deworming behaviour and lifestyle of pets associated with the risk of endoparasites. Parasit. Vectors 12, 480.

Saiki, R.K., Scharf, S., Faloona, F., Mullis, K.B., Horn, G.T., Erlich, H.A., Arnheim, N., 1985. Enzymatic amplification of β-globin genomic sequences and restriction site analysis for diagnosis of sickle cell anemia. Science (New York, *N.Y.)* 230, 1350–1354.

Saiki, R., Gyllensten, U., Erlich, H., 1988. The polymerase chain reaction. In: Genome Analysis: A Practical Approach.

Salazar, G., Russi-Vigoya, M.N., 2021. Technology readiness level as the Foundation of Human Readiness Level. Ergon. Des. 29 (4), 25–29.

Sallé, G., Cortet, J., Bois, I., Dubès, C., Guyot-Sionest, Q., Larrieu, C., Landrin, V., Majorel, G., Wittreck, S., Woringer, E., Couroucé, A., Guillot, J., Jacquiet, P., Guégnard, F., Blanchard, A., Leblond, A., 2017. Risk factor analysis of equine strongyle resistance to anthelmintics. Int. J. Parasitol. Drugs Drug Resist. 7 (3), 407–415.

Sanchez, J., Dohoo, I.R., Markham, F., Leslie, K., Conboy, G., 2002. Evaluation of the repeatability of a crude adult indirect *Ostertagia ostertagi* ELISA and methods of expressing test results. Vet. Parasitol. 109 (1–2), 75–90.

Santos, M.C., Redman, E., Amarante, M.R.V., Gilleard, J.S., Amarante, A.F.T., 2017. A panel of microsatellite markers to discriminate and study interactions between *Haemonchus contortus* and *Haemonchus placei*. Vet. Parasitol. 244, 71–75.

Sapp, S.G.H., Elsemore, D.A., Hanna, R., Yabsley, M.J., 2020. Experimental comparison of *Baylisascaris procyonis* definitive host competence between domestic dogs and raccoons (*Procyon lotor*). Parasitology 147, 1344–1351.

Sargison, N.D., Redman, E., Morrison, A.A., Bartley, D.J., Jackson, F., Naghra-van Gijzel, H., Holroyd, N., Berriman, M., Cotton, J.A., Gilleard, J.S., 2018. A method for single pair mating in an obligate parasitic nematode. Int. J. Parasitol. 48, 159–165.

Sargison, N.D., MacLeay, M., Morrison, A.A., Bartley, D.J., Evans, M., Chaudhry, U., 2019a. Development of amplicon sequencing for the analysis of benzimidazole resistance allele frequencies in field populations of gastrointestinal nematodes. Int. J. Parasitol. Drugs Drug Resist. 10, 92–100.

Sargison, N.D., Redman, E., Morrison, A.A., Bartley, D.J., Jackson, F., Hoberg, E., Gilleard, J.S., 2019b. Mating barriers between genetically divergent strains of the parasitic nematode *Haemonchus contortus* suggest incipient speciation. Int. J. Parasitol. 49, 531–540.

Scala, A., Tamponi, A., Sanna, G., Predieri, G., Meloni, L., Knoll, S., Sedda, G., Dessì, G., Cappai, M.G., Varcasia, A., 2022. *Parascaris* spp. eggs in horses of Italy: a large-scale epidemiological analysis of the egg excretion and conditioning factors. Front. Vet. Sci. 10 (9), 892920.

Scare, J.A., Slusarewicz, P., Noel, M.L., Wielgus, K.M., Nielsen, M.K., 2017. Evaluation of accuracy and precision of a smartphone based automated parasite egg counting system in comparison to the McMaster and mini-FLOTAC methods. Vet. Parasitol. 247, 85–92.

Scare, J.A., Steuer, A.E., Gravatte, H.S., Kálmán, C., Ramires, L., Dias de Castro, L.L., Norris, J.K., Miller, F., Camargo, F., Lawyer, A., De Pedro, P., Jolly, B., Nielsen, M.K., 2018. Management practices associated with strongylid parasite prevalence on horse farms in rural counties of Kentucky. Vet. Parasitol.: Reg. Stud. Rep. 14, 25–31.

Schloss, P.D., Westcott, S.L., Ryabin, T., Hall, J.R., Hartmann, M., Hollister, E.B., Lesniewski, R.A., Oakley, B.B., Parks, D.H., Robinson, C.J., Sahl, J.W., Stres, B., Thallinger, G.G., Van Horn, D.J., Weber, C.F., 2009. Introducing mothur: open-source, platform-independent, community-supported software for describing and comparing microbial communities. Appl. Environ. Microbiol. 75, 7537–7541.

Schwenkenbecher, J.M., Kaplan, R.M., 2009. Real-time PCR assays for monitoring benzimidazole resistance-associated mutations in *Ancylostoma caninum*. Exp. Parasitol. 122, 6–10.

Schwenkenbecher, J.M., Albonico, M., Bickle, Q., Kaplan, R.M., 2007. Characterization of beta-tubulin genes in hookworms and investigation of resistance-associated mutations using real-time PCR. Mol. Biochem. Parasitol. 156, 167–174.

Scott, H., Gilleard, J.S., Jelinski, M., Barkema, H.W., Redman, E.M., Avramenko, R.W., Luby, C., Kelton, D.F., Bauman, C.A., Keefe, G., Dubuc, J., Uehlinger, F.D., 2019. Prevalence, fecal egg counts, and species identification of gastrointestinal nematodes in replacement dairy heifers in Canada. J. Dairy Sci. 102, 8251–8263.

Seesao, Y., Gay, M., Merlin, S., Viscogliosi, E., Aliouat-Denis, C.M., Audebert, C., 2017. A review of methods for nematode identification. J. Microbiol. Methods 138, 37–49.

Shaw, R.J., Morris, C.A., Wheeler, M., Tate, M., Sutherland, I.A., 2012. Salivary IgA: a suitable measure of immunity to gastrointestinal nematodes in sheep. Vet. Parasitol. 186 (1–2), 109–117.

Shaw, R.J., Morris, C.A., Wheeler, M., 2013. Genetic and phenotypic relationships between carbohydrate larval antigen (CarLA) IgA, parasite resistance and productivity in serial samples taken from lambs after weaning. Int. J. Parasitol. 43 (8), 661–667.

Sheka, D., Alabi, N., Gordon, P.M.K., 2021. Oxford nanopore sequencing in clinical microbiology and infection diagnostics. Brief. Bioinform. 22 (bbaa403).

Shiraho, E.A., Eric, A.L., Mwangi, I.N., Maina, G.M., Kinuthia, J.M., Mutuku, M.W., Mugambi, R.M., Mwandi, J.M., Mkoji, G.M., 2016. Development of a loop mediated isothermal amplification for diagnosis of Ascaris lumbricoides in fecal samples. J. Parasitol. Res. 2016 (7376207).

Sidstedt, M., Rådström, P., Hedman, J., 2020. PCR inhibition in qPCR, dPCR and MPS—mechanisms and solutions. Anal. Bioanal. Chem. 412, 2009–2023.

Silvestre, A., Cabaret, J., 2002. Mutation in position 167 of isotype 1 beta-tubulin gene of Trichostrongylid nematodes: role in benzimidazole resistance? Mol. Biochem. Parasitol. 120, 297–300.

Singh, B., Flampouri, E., Dempsey, E., 2019. Electrochemical enzyme-linked immunosorbent assay (e-ELISA) for parasitic nematode: *Ostertagia ostertagi* (brown stomach worm) infections in dairy cattle. Analyst 144 (19), 5748–5754.

Skuce, P., Stenhouse, L., Jackson, F., Hypša, V., Gilleard, J., 2010. Benzimidazole resistance allele haplotype diversity in United Kingdom isolates of *Teladorsagia circumcincta* supports a hypothesis of multiple origins of resistance by recurrent mutation. Int. J. Parasitol. 40, 1247–1255.

Slusarewicz, P., Pagano, S., Mills, C., Popa, G., Chow, K.M., Mendenhall, M., Rodgers, D.W., Nielsen, M.K., 2016. Automated parasite faecal egg counting using fluorescence labelling, smartphone image capture and computational image analysis. Int. J. Parasitol. 46 (8), 485–493.

Slusarewicz, M., Slusarewicz, P., Nielsen, M.K., 2019. The effect of counting duration on quantitative fecal egg count test performance. Vet. Parasitol.: X 2, 100020.

Slusarewicz, P., Slusarewicz, J.H., Nielsen, M.K., 2021. Development and performance of an automated fecal egg count system for small ruminant strongylids. Vet. Parasitol. 295, 109442.

Sobotyk, C., Upton, K.E., Lejeune, M., Nolan, T.J., Marsh, A.E., Herrin, B.H., Borst, M.M., Piccione, J., Zajac, A.M., Camp, L.E., Pulaski, C.N., Starkey, L.A., von Simson, C., Verocai, G.G., 2021. Retrospective study of canine endoparasites diagnosed by fecal flotation methods analyzed across veterinary parasitology diagnostic laboratories, United States, 2018. Parasit. Vectors 14 (1), 439.

Sommer, C., 1996. Digital image analysis and identification of eggs from bovine parasitic nematodes. J. Helminthol. 70 (2), 143–151.

Sommer, C., 1998. Quantitative characterization of texture used for identification of eggs of bovine parasitic nematodes. J. Helminthol. 72 (2), 179–182.

Stafford, K., Kollasch, T.M., Duncan, K.T., Horr, S., Goddu, T., Heinz-Loomer, C., Rumschlag, A.J., Ryan, W.G., Sweet, S., Little, S.E., 2020. Detection of gastrointestinal parasitism at recreational canine sites in the USA: the DOGPARCS study. Parasit. Vectors 13 (1), 1–10.

Stanley, K.K., Szewczuk, E., 2005. Multiplexed tandem PCR: gene profiling from small amounts of RNA using SYBR Green detection. Nucleic Acids Res. 33, e180.

Stoll, N.R., 1923. Investigations on the control of hookworm disease. XV. An effective method of counting hookworm eggs in faeces. Am. J. Epidemiol. 3, 59–70.

Stoll, N.R., 1930. On methods of counting nematode ova in sheep dung. Parasitology 22, 116–136.

Stracke, K., Clarke, N., Awburn, C.V., Nery, S.V., Khieu, V., Traub, R.J., Jex, A.R., 2019. Development and validation of a multiplexed-tandem qPCR tool for diagnostics of human soil-transmitted helminth infections. PLoS Negl. Trop. Dis. 13, e0007363.

Strube, C., Neubert, A., Springer, A., von Samson-Himmelstjerna, G., 2019. Survey of German pet owners quantifying endoparasitic infection risk and implications for deworming recommendations. Parasit. Vectors 12, 203.

Stuyver, L.J., Levecke, B., 2021. The role of diagnostic technologies to measure progress toward WHO 2030 targets for soil-transmitted helminth control programs. PLoS Negl. Trop. Dis. 15 (6), e0009422.

Sukas, S., Van Dorst, B., Kryj, A., Lagatie, O., De Malsche, W., Stuyver, L.J., 2019. Development of a lab-on-a-disk platform with digital imaging for identification and counting of parasite eggs in human and animal stool. Micromachines 10 (12), 852.

Suzuki, C.T.N., Gomes, J.F., Falcão, A.X., Hoshino-Shimizu, S., Papa, J.P., 2013. Automated diagnosis of human intestinal parasites using optical microscopy images. In: *Proceedings of the IEEE 10th International Symposium on Biomedical Imaging, San Francisco, CA, USA, 7–11 April 2013*, pp. 460–463.

Sweet, S., Hegarty, E., McCrann, D.J., Coyne, M., Kincaid, D., Szlosek, D., 2021. A 3-year retrospective analysis of canine intestinal parasites: fecal testing positivity by age, U.S. geographical region and reason for veterinary visit. Parasit. Vectors 14 (1), 1–9.

Sykes, A.M., McCarthy, J.S., 2011. A coproantigen diagnostic test for *Strongyloides* infection. PLoS Negl. Trop. Dis. 5, e955.

Taniuchi, M., Verweij, J.J., Noor, Z., Sobuz, S.U., Van Lieshout, L., Petri, W.A., Haque, R., Houpt, E.R., 2011. High throughput multiplex PCR and probe-based detection with luminex beads for seven intestinal parasites. Am. J. Trop. Med. Hyg. 84, 332–337.

Tarbiat, B., Enweji, N., Baltrusis, P., Halvarsson, P., Osterman-Lind, E., Jansson, D.S., Höglund, J., 2021. A novel duplex ddPCR assay for detection and differential diagnosis of *Ascaridia galli* and *Heterakis gallinarum* eggs from chickens feces. Vet. Parasitol. 296, 109499.

Taskin, B., Gozen, A.G., Duran, M., 2011. Selective quantification of viable *Escherichia coli* bacteria in biosolids by quantitative PCR with propidium monoazide modification. Appl. Environ. Microbiol. 77, 4329–4335.

Taylor, M.A., 2012. SCOPS and COWS- -'worming it out of UK farmers. Vet. Parasitol. 186, 65–69.

Tekin, K., Begüm Yurdakok-Dikmen, B., Kanca, H., Guatteo, R., 2021. Precision livestock farming technologies: novel direction of information flow. Ank. Univ. Vet. Fak. Derg. 68, 193–212.

Temperley, N.D., Webster, L.M.I., Adam, A., Keller, L.F., Johnson, P.C.D., 2009. Cross-species utility of microsatellite markers in trichostrongyloid nematodes. J. Parasitol. 95, 487–489.

Teoli, D., Sanvictores, T., An, J., 2021. SWOT analysis. In: StatPearls. StatPearls Publishing.

Thakur, S., Hill, D., Susick, E., 2013. Similarities in seroprevalence of *toxoplasma gondii, trichinella* spp., *Trichuris suis* and *Ascaris suum* in swine in the conventional and antibiotic free swine production systems. In: Proceedings of Safepork, pp. 133–136.

Thamsborg, S.M., Ketzis, J., Horii, Y., Matthews, J.B., 2017. Strongyloides spp. infections of veterinary importance. Parasitology 144, 274–284.

Thienpont, D., Rochette, F., Vanparijs, O.F.J., 1986. Diagnosing Helminthiasis by Coprological Examination, second ed. Janssen Research Foundation, Beerse.

Toaleb, N.I., Abdel-Rahman, E.H., 2021. Potentials of glycoprotein fraction in successful diagnosis of sheep haemonchosis. Adv. Anim. Vet. Sci. 9 (3), 335–343.

Tombak, K.J., Budischak, S.A., Hauck, S., Martinez, L.A., Rubenstein, D.I., 2020. The non-invasive measurement of faecal immunoglobulin in African equids. Int. J. Parasitol. Parasites Wildl. 12, 105–112.

Torres-Sangiao, E., Leal Rodriguez, C., García-Riestra, C., 2021. Application and perspectives of MALDI-TOF mass spectrometry in clinical microbiology laboratories. Microorganisms 9, 1539.
Traversa, D., 2011. Are we paying too much attention to cardio-pulmonary nematodes and neglecting old-fashioned worms like *Trichuris vulpis*? Parasit. Vectors 4 (1), 32.
Traversa, D., 2012. Pet roundworms and hookworms: A continuing need for global worming. Parasit. Vectors 5, 91.
Troell, K., Mattsson, J.G., Alderborn, A., Höglund, J., 2003. Pyrosequencing™ analysis identifies discrete populations of *Haemonchus contortus* from small ruminants. Int. J. Parasitol. 33, 765–771.
Troell, K., Engström, A., Morrison, D.A., Mattsson, J.G., Höglund, J., 2006. Global patterns reveal strong population structure in *Haemonchus contortus*, a nematode parasite of domesticated ruminants. Int. J. Parasitol. 36, 1305–1316.
Tröger, V., Niemann, K., Gärting, C., Kuhlmeier, D., 2015. Isothermal amplification and quantification of nucleic acids and its use in microsystems. J. Nanomed. Nanotechnol. 06.
Tyson, F., Dalesman, S., Brophy, P.M., Morphew, R.M., 2020. Novel equine Faecal egg diagnostics: validation of the FECPAK^{G2}. Animals 10 (8), 1254.
Tzelos, T., Geyer, K.K., Mitchell, M.C., McWilliam, H.E.G., Kharchenko, V.O., Burgess, S.T.G., Matthews, J.B., 2020. Characterisation of serum IgG(T) responses to potential diagnostic antigens for equine cyathostominosis. Int. J. Parasitol. 50 (4), 289–298.
van der Voort, M., Charlier, J., Lauwers, L., Vercruysse, J., Van Huylenbroeck, G., Van Meensel, J., 2013. Conceptual framework for analysing farm-specific economic effects of helminth infections in ruminants and control strategies. Prev. Vet. Med. 109, 228–235.
Vandekerckhove, E., Vlaminck, J., Geldhof, P., 2017. Evaluation of serology to measure exposure of piglets to *ascaris suum* during the nursery phase. Vet. Parasitol. 246, 82–87.
Vandekerckhove, E., Vlaminck, J., del Pozo Sacristán, R., Geldhof, P., 2019. Effect of strategic deworming on *ascaris suum* exposure and technical performance parameters in fattening pigs. Vet. Parasitol. 268, 67–72.
Vanderstichel, R., Dohoo, I., Sanchez, J., Sithole, F., Keefe, G., Stryhn, H., 2013. Predicting the effect of anthelmintic treatment on milk production of dairy cattle in Canada using an *Ostertagia ostertagi* ELISA from individual milk samples. Prev. Vet. Med. 111 (1–2), 63–75.
Vercruysse, J., Charlier, J., Van Dijk, J., Morgan, E.R., Geary, T., von Samson-Himmelstjerna, G., Claerebout, E., 2018. Control of helminth ruminant infections by 2030. Parasitology 145 (13), 1655–1664.
Verweij, J.J., Brienen, E.A.T., Ziem, J., Yelifari, L., Polderman, A.M., Van Lieshout, L., 2007. Simultaneous detection and quantification of *Ancylostoma duodenale*, *Necator americanus*, and *Oesophagostomum bifurcum* in fecal samples using multiplex real-time PCR. Am. J. Trop. Med. Hyg. 77, 685–690.
Verweij, J.J., Canales, M., Polman, K., Ziem, J., Brienen, E.A.T., Polderman, A.M., van Lieshout, L., 2009. Molecular diagnosis of *Strongyloides stercoralis* in faecal samples using real-time PCR. Trans. R. Soc. Trop. Med. Hyg. 103, 342–346.
Villa-Mancera, A., Pastelín-Rojas, C., Olivares-Pérez, J., Córdova-Izquierdo, A., Reynoso-Palomar, A., 2018. Bulk tank milk prevalence and production losses, spatial analysis, and predictive risk mapping of *Ostertagia ostertagi* infections in Mexican cattle herds. Parasitol. Res. 117 (5), 1613–1620.
Vlaminck, J., Martinez-Valladares, M., Dewilde, S., Moens, L., Tilleman, K., Deforce, D., Urban, J., Claerebout, E., Vercruysse, J., Geldhof, P., 2011. Immunizing pigs with *ascaris suum* haemoglobin increases the inflammatory response in the liver but fails to induce a protective immunity. Parasite Immunol. 33 (4), 250–254.

Vlaminck, J., Nejsum, P., Vangroenweghe, F., Thamsborg, S.M., Vercruysse, J., Geldhof, P., 2012. Evaluation of a serodiagnostic test using *ascaris suum* haemoglobin for the detection of roundworm infections in pig populations. Vet. Parasitol. 189 (2–4), 267–273.

Vlaminck, J., Düsseldorf, S., Heres, L., Geldhof, P., 2015. Serological examination of fattening pigs reveals associations between *ascaris suum*, lung pathogens and technical performance parameters. Vet. Parasitol. 210 (3–4), 151–158.

Vlaminck, J., Masure, D., Wang, T., Nejsum, P., Hokke, C.H., Geldhof, P., 2016. A phosphorylcholine-containing glycolipid-like antigen present on the surface of infective stage larvae of *ascaris* spp. is a major antibody target in infected pigs and humans. PLoS Negl. Trop. Dis. 10 (12), 1–20.

Vlaminck, J., Cools, P., Albonico, M., Ame, S., Ayana, M., Cringoli, G., Dana, D., Keiser, J., Maurelli, M.P., Matoso, L.F., Montresor, A., Mekonnen, Z., Mirams, G., Corrêa-Oliveira, R., Pinto, S.A., Rinaldi, L., Sayasone, S., Thomas, E., Vercruysse, J., Verweij, J.J., Levecke, B., 2019. Therapeutic efficacy of albendazole against soil-transmitted helminthiasis in children measured by five diagnostic methods. PLoS Negl. Trop. Dis. 13 (8), e0007471.

von Samson-Himmelstjerna, G., 2006. Molecular diagnosis of anthelmintic resistance. Vet. Parasitol. 136, 99–107.

von Samson-Himmelstjerna, G., Harder, A., Schnieder, T., 2002. Quantitative analysis of ITS2 sequences in trichostrongyle parasites. Int. J. Parasitol. 32, 1529–1535.

von Samson-Himmelstjerna, G., Buschbaum, S., Wirtherle, N., Pape, M., Schnieder, T., 2003. TaqMan minor groove binder real-time PCR analysis of β-tubulin codon 200 polymorphism in small strongyles (cyathostomin) indicates that the TAC allele is only moderately selected in benzimidazole-resistant populations. Parasitology 127, 489–496.

von Samson-Himmelstjerna, G., Walsh, T.K., Donnan, A.A., Carrière, S., Jackson, F., Skuce, P.J., Rohn, K., Wolstenholme, A.J., 2009. Molecular detection of benzimidazole resistance in *Haemonchus contortus* using real-time PCR and pyrosequencing. Parasitology 136, 349–358.

Walsh, T.K., Donnan, A.A., Jackson, F., Skuce, P., Wolstenholme, A.J., 2007. Detection and measurement of benzimidazole resistance alleles in *Haemonchus contortus* using real-time PCR with locked nucleic acid Taqman probes. Vet. Parasitol. 144, 304–312.

Walshe, N., Mulcahy, G., Crispie, F., Cabrera-Rubio, R., Cotter, P., Jahns, H., Duggan, V., 2021. Outbreak of acute larval cyathostominosis – A "perfect storm" of inflammation and dysbiosis. Equine Vet. J. 53 (4), 727–739.

Wang, Y., Prosen, D.E., Mei, L., Sullivan, J.C., Finney, M., Vander Horn, P.B., 2004. A novel strategy to engineer DNA polymerases for enhanced processivity and improved performance *in vitro*. Nucleic Acids Res. 32, 1197–1207.

Wang, C.R., Gao, J.F., Zhu, X.Q., Zhao, Q., 2012a. Characterization of *Bunostomum trigonocephalum* and *Bunostomum phlebotomum* from sheep and cattle by internal transcribed spacers of nuclear ribosomal DNA. Res. Vet. Sci. 92, 99–102.

Wang, J.X., Pan, C.S., Cui, L.W., 2012b. Application of a real-time PCR method for detecting and monitoring hookworm *Necator americanus* infections in southern China. Asian Pac. J. Trop. Biomed. 2, 925–929.

Wang, X.-C., Liu, C., Huang, L., Bengtsson-Palme, J., Chen, H., Zhang, J.H., Cai, D., Li, J.Q., 2015. ITS1: a DNA barcode better than ITS2 in eukaryotes? Mol. Ecol. Resour. 15, 573–586.

Wang, T., Avramenko, R.W., Redman, E.M., Wit, J., Gilleard, J.S., Colwell, D.D., 2020. High levels of third-stage larvae (L3) overwinter survival for multiple cattle gastrointestinal nematode species on western Canadian pastures as revealed by ITS2 rDNA metabarcoding. Parasit. Vectors 13, 458.

Wang, T., Redman, E.M., Morosetti, A., Chen, R., Kulle, S., Morden, N., McFarland, C., Vineer, H.R., Colwell, D.D., Morgan, E.R., Gilleard, J.S., 2021. Seasonal epidemiology of gastrointestinal nematodes of cattle in the northern continental climate zone of western Canada as revealed by internal transcribed spacer-2 ribosomal DNA nemabiome barcoding. Parasit. Vectors 14, 604.

Watts, M.R., James, G., Sultana, Y., Ginn, A.N., Outhred, A.C., Kong, F., Verweij, J.J., Iredell, J.R., Chen, S.C.A., Lee, R., 2014. A loop-mediated isothermal amplification (LAMP) assay for *Strongyloides stercoralis* in stool that uses a visual detection method with SYTO-82 fluorescent dye. Am. J. Trop. Med. Hyg. 90, 306–311.

Watts, M.R., Kim, R., Ahuja, V., Robertson, G.J., Sultana, Y., Wehrhahn, M.C., Bradbury, R.S., Gilbert, G.L., Lee, R., 2018. Comparison of loop-mediated isothermal amplification and real-time PCR assays for detection of strongyloides larvae in different specimen matrices. J. Clin. Microbiol. 57. e01173-18.

WHO, 2021. Diagnostic Target Product Profile for Monitoring and Evaluation of Soil-Transmitted Helminth Control Programmes. Geneva, Switzerland.

Williams, E.G., Brophy, P.M., Williams, H.W., Davies, N., Jones, R.A., 2021. Gastrointestinal nematode control practices in ewes: identification of factors associated with application of control methods known to influence anthelmintic resistance development. Vet. Parasitol.: Reg. Stud. Rep. 24, 100562.

Wittwer, C.T., 2009. High-resolution DNA melting analysis: advancements and limitations. Hum. Mutat. 30, 857–859.

Wittwer, C.T., Reed, G.H., Gundry, C.N., Vandersteen, J.G., Pryor, R.J., 2003. High-resolution genotyping by amplicon melting analysis using LCGreen. Clin. Chem. 49 (6 Pt 1), 853–860.

Wong, Y.P., Othman, S., Lau, Y.L., Radu, S., Chee, H.Y., 2018. Loop-mediated isothermal amplification (LAMP): a versatile technique for detection of micro-organisms. J. Appl. Microbiol. 124 (3), 626–643.

Workentine, M.L., Chen, R., Zhu, S., Gavriliuc, S., Shaw, N., de Rijke, J., Redman, E.M., Avramenko, R.W., Wit, J., Poissant, J., Gilleard, J.S., 2020. A database for ITS2 sequences from nematodes. BMC Genet. 21, 74.

Xia, Y., Gu, H.F., Peng, R., Chen, Q., Zheng, Y.C., Murphy, R.W., Zeng, X.M., 2012. COI is better than 16S rRNA for DNA barcoding Asiatic salamanders (amphibia: Caudata: Hynobiidae). Mol. Ecol. Resour. 12, 48–56.

Xu, J., 2016. Fungal DNA barcoding. Genome 59, 913–932.

Yang, X., Qi, M.W., Zhang, Z.Z., Gao, C., Wang, C.Q., Lei, W.Q., Tan, L., Zhao, J.L., Fang, R., Hu, M., 2017. Development and evaluation of a loop-mediated isothermal amplification (lamp) assay for the detection of *Haemonchus contortus* in goat fecal samples. J. Parasitol. 103, 161–167.

Yoon, E.J., Jeong, S.H., 2021. MALDI-TOF mass spectrometry technology as a tool for the rapid diagnosis of antimicrobial resistance in bacteria. Antibiotics (Basel, Switzerland) 10, 982.

Yu, Z., Zhao, Z., Chen, L., Li, J., Ju, X., 2020. Development of a droplet digital PCR for detection of Trichuriasis in sheep. J. Parasitol. 106, 603–610.

Zajac, A.M., Conboy, G.A., 2012. Veterinary Clinical Parasitology, eighth ed. Blackwell Publishing, Ames, Iowa, p. 368.

Zajac, A.M., Garza, J., 2020. Biology, epidemiology, and control of gastrointestinal nematodes of small ruminants. *The veterinary clinics of North America.* Food Anim. Pract. 36, 73–87.

Zarlenga, D.S., Stringfellow, F., Nobary, M., Lichtenfels, J.R., 1994. Cloning and characterization of ribosomal RNA genes from three species of *Haemonchus* (Nematoda: Trichostrongyloidea) and identification of PCR primers for rapid differentiation. Exp. Parasitol. 78, 28–36.

Zarlenga, D.S., Gasbarre, L.C., Boyd, P., Leighton, E., Lichtenfels, J.R., 1998a. Identification and semi-quantitation of *Ostertagia ostertagi* eggs by enzymatic amplification of ITS-1 sequences. Vet. Parasitol. 77, 245–257.

Zarlenga, D.S., Hoberg, E.P., Stringfellow, F., Lichtenfels, J.R., 1998b. Comparisons of two polymorphic species of *Ostertagia* and phylogenetic relationships within the Ostertagiinae (Nematoda: Trichostrongyloidea) inferred from ribosomal DNA repeat and mitochondrial DNA sequences. J. Parasitol. 84, 806–812.

Zhan, B., Liu, Y., Badamchian, M., Williamson, A., Feng, J., Loukas, A., Hawdon, J.M., Hotez, P.J., 2003. Molecular characterisation of the *Ancylostoma*-secreted protein family from the adult stage of *Ancylostoma caninum*. Int. J. Parasitol. 33 (9), 897–907.

Zhao, G.H., Jia, Y.Q., Bian, Q.Q., Nisbet, A.J., Cheng, W.Y., Liu, Y., Fang, Y.Q., Ma, X.T., Yu, S.K., 2015. Molecular approaches to differentiate three species of *Nematodirus* in sheep and goats from China based on internal transcribed spacer rDNA sequences. J. Helminthol. 89, 259–266.

Zheng, Y., Xie, Y., Geldhof, P., Vlaminck, J., Ma, G., Gasser, R.B., Wang, T., 2020. High anti-*ascaris* seroprevalence in fattening pigs in Sichuan, China, calls for improved management strategies. Parasit. Vectors 13 (1), 60.

Zhou, L., Errigo, R.J., Lu, H., Poritz, M.A., Seipp, M.T., Wittwer, C.T., 2008. Snapback primer genotyping with saturating DNA dye and melting analysis. Clin. Chem. 54, 1648–1656.

Zhu, X.Q., Jacobs, D.E., Chilton, N.B., Sani, R.A., Cheng, N.A.B.Y., Gasser, R.B., 1998. Molecular characterization of a *Toxocara* variant from cats in Kuala Lumpur, Malaysia. Parasitology 117, 155–164.

FSC
www.fsc.org
MIX
Papier | Fördert gute Waldnutzung
FSC® C083411

Kolibri 360 GmbH
Ferdinand-Jühlke-Straße 7
99095 Erfurt, Deutschland
produktsicherheit@kolibri360.de